Second Edition

Appleton & Lange Review of
Pharmacology

MW00685528

Joseph J. Krzanowski, Jr., PhD
Professor and Associate Dean
Department of Pharmacology and Therapeutics
College of Medicine
University of South Florida
Tampa, Florida

James B. Polson, PhD
Professor
Department of Pharmacology and Therapeutics
College of Medicine
University of South Florida
Tampa, Florida

Appleton & Lange Reviews/McGraw-Hill
Medical Publishing Division

New York   Chicago   San Francisco   Lisbon   London   Madrid   Mexico City   Milan
New Delhi   San Juan   Seoul   Singapore   Sydney   Toronto

McGraw-Hill

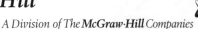

A Division of The McGraw-Hill Companies

Notice

Medicine is an ever-changing science. As new research and clinical experience broaden our knowledge, changes in treatment and drug therapy are required. The authors and the publisher of this work have checked with sources believed to be reliable in their efforts to provide information that is complete and generally in accord with the standards accepted at the time of publication. However, in view of the possibility of human error or changes in medical sciences, neither the authors nor the publisher nor any other party who has been involved in the preparation or publication of this work warrants that the information contained herein is in every respect accurate or complete, and they disclaim all responsibility for any errors or omissions or for the results obtained from use of such information contained in this work. Readers are encouraged to confirm the information contained herein with other sources. For example and in particular, readers are advised to check the product information sheet included in the package of each drug they plan to administer to be certain that the information contained in this work is accurate and that changes have not been made in the recommended dose or in the contraindications for administration. This recommendation is of particular importance in connection with new or infrequently used drugs.

This book was set in Palatino by Rainbow Graphics.
The editors were Catherine A. Johnson and John M. Morriss.
The production supervisor was Lisa Mendez.
Von Hoffman Graphics was printer and binder.

This book was printed on acid-free paper.

Library of Congress Cataloging-in-Publication Data
Krzanowski, Joseph J.
Appleton & Lange review of pharmacology/Joseph J. Krzanowski, Jr., James B. Polson.
  p. ; cm.
  Includes bibliographical references.
  ISBN 0-07-137743-3 (alk. paper)
   1. Pharmacology—Examinations, questions, etc. I. Title: Appleton and Lange review
of pharmacology. II. Title: Review of pharmacology. III. Polson, James B. IV. Title.
  [DNLM: 1. Pharmaceutical Preparations—Examination Questions 2.
Pharmacology—Examination Questions. QV 18.2 K94a 2002]
RM301.13 .K797 2002
615'.1'076—dc21   2002026556

Contents

CHAPTER 1

Principles of Pharmacology
Questions

DIRECTIONS (Questions 1 through 53): Each of the numbered items or incomplete statements in this section is followed by answers or by completions of the statement. Select the ONE lettered answer or completion that is BEST in each case.

1. Chirality (stereoisomerism) is common among drugs, and therefore many drugs exist as enantiomeric pairs. Which of the following characteristic(s) of drugs is (are) commonly affected by chirality?

   (A) the ability of the drug to activate its receptor
   (B) the affinity of the drug's binding to its receptor site
   (C) the goodness of fit of the drug into its receptor site
   (D) the rate of metabolism of the drug by drug-metabolizing enzymes
   (E) all of the above

2. Drugs bind to their target receptors by means of chemical forces or bonds. Of the following bond types, which is least likely to contribute to very selective drug action?

   (A) covalent bonds
   (B) hydrogen bonds
   (C) hydrophobic bonds
   (D) ionic bonds
   (E) van der Waals forces

3. Which of the following types of drugs binds to a receptor site but does not produce any direct pharmacological effect?

   (A) agonist
   (B) antagonist
   (C) inverse agonist
   (D) inverse partial agonist
   (E) partial agonist

4. Of the processes by which drugs are distributed throughout the body, which of the following is most dependent on the ability of a drug to dissolve in a lipid medium?

   (A) transport by diffusion across aqueous compartments
   (B) transport by diffusion across membranes
   (C) transport by endocytosis
   (D) transport by exocytosis
   (E) transport by special carriers

5. The passive flux of drug molecules is given by Fick's law. Which of the following factors is not included in the calculation of flux by this method?

   (A) the area across which diffusion is occurring
   (B) the concentration gradient across the path
   (C) the density of the medium
   (D) the length of the path
   (E) the permeability coefficient of the drug

6. Which of the following types of amines is (are) permanently charged?

   (A) primary
   (B) quarternary
   (C) secondary
   (D) tertiary
   (E) all of the above

7. A patient has ingested toxic amounts of aspirin, which is a weak acid. Which of the following measures can increase the excretion of aspirin in the urine?

   (A) administration of a weak base
   (B) administration of ammonium chloride
   (C) administration of ascorbic acid
   (D) administration of sodium bicarbonate
   (E) none of the above

8. Which of the following equations can be used to calculate the degree of ionization of weak acids and weak bases?

   (A) the equation for zero-order processes
   (B) the Fick equation
   (C) the Henderson–Hasselbalch equation
   (D) the Michaelis–Menten equation
   (E) the Schild equation

9. Theophylline is a weak acid with a pK_a equal to 8.8. What will be the ratio of un-ionized/ionized forms at a pH equal to 7.8?

   (A) 1/100
   (B) 1/10
   (C) 1/1
   (D) 10/1
   (E) 100/1

10. Which of the following factors determine(s) whether a drug will bind to a particular receptor and with what avidity?

    (A) the drug's electrical charge
    (B) the drug's molecular shape
    (C) the drug's molecular size
    (D) all of the above
    (E) none of the above

11. Which of the following types of macromolecules is targeted by cardioactive digitalis glycosides to produce their pharmacological effects on the heart?

    (A) enzymes
    (B) nucleic acids
    (C) regulatory proteins, which are receptors for endogenous ligands such as neurotransmitters, autacoids, and hormones
    (D) structural proteins
    (E) transport proteins

12. Which of the following characteristics of drug-receptor interactions is the reciprocal of the equilibrium dissociation constant (K_D)?

    (A) affinity
    (B) EC_{50}
    (C) efficacy
    (D) intrinsic activity
    (E) maximum binding

13. In idealized or in vitro systems, the relationship between drug concentration and effect is best described by what kind of curve?

    (A) hyperbolic
    (B) linear
    (C) parabolic
    (D) sigmoidal
    (E) none of the above

14. What is the typical effect of a reversible, competitive antagonist on an agonist concentration-effect curve?

    (A) It will decrease the EC_{50} but not change the maximum effect.
    (B) It will decrease the EC_{50} and decrease the maximum effect.
    (C) It will increase the EC_{50} but not change the maximum effect.
    (D) It will increase the EC_{50} and decrease the maximum effect.
    (E) It will not affect the EC_{50}, but it will decrease the maximum effect.

15. In a tissue that does not have "spare" receptors, what is the typical effect of an irreversible antagonist on an agonist concentration-response curve?

   (A) It will decrease the EC_{50} but not change the maximum effect.
   (B) It will decrease the EC_{50} and decrease the maximum effect.
   (C) It will increase the EC_{50} but not change the maximum effect.
   (D) It will increase the EC_{50} and decrease the maximum effect.
   (E) It will not affect the EC_{50}, but it will decrease the maximum effect.

16. A physician may use protamine to reverse the anticoagulant effects of heparin. This is an example of what kind of antagonism?

   (A) allosteric
   (B) chemical
   (C) competitive
   (D) irreversible
   (E) physiological

17. A physician may use insulin to counteract the hyperglycemic effects of glucocorticoids. This is an example of what kind of antagonism?

   (A) allosteric
   (B) chemical
   (C) competitive
   (D) irreversible
   (E) physiological

18. "Desensitization" of the beta-adrenoceptor in the continued presence of an agonist is most likely associated with

   (A) decreased receptor biosynthesis
   (B) decreased receptor recycling
   (C) receptor downregulation
   (D) receptor internalization
   (E) receptor phosphorylation

19. Which of the following pharmacological terms is most closely related to the relative position of a graded dose-response curve on the dose or concentration axis, that is, the ED_{50} or EC_{50}?

   (A) efficacy
   (B) intrinsic activity
   (C) potency
   (D) specificity
   (E) variability

20. Which of the following effects best lends itself to analysis by quantal dose-effect curves?

   (A) conversion of cardiac arrhythmias to normal rhythms in a patient population
   (B) increasing the contractile force of a failing heart
   (C) increasing urinary excretion of sodium in a patient with congestive heart failure
   (D) lowering of blood pressure in a patient with hypertension
   (E) the relaxation of a respiratory smooth muscle preparation in an isolated tissue bath

21. A ratio that relates the desired effect of a drug to an undesired effect is the ratio of the TD_{50} to the ED_{50}. By what pharmacological term is this ratio known?

   (A) effective dose ratio
   (B) median effective dose
   (C) median toxic dose
   (D) pharmacological efficacy
   (E) therapeutic index

22. Which of the following terms refers to an unusual drug response, that is, one that is infrequently observed in most patients?

   (A) hyperreactive response
   (B) hyporeactive response
   (C) idiosyncratic response
   (D) tachyphylaxis
   (E) tolerance

23. What is the pharmacological term that refers to the rapid diminution of a tissue's sensitivity to a drug after administration?

    (A) hypersensitivity
    (B) hyporeactivity
    (C) idiosyncrasy
    (D) tachyphylaxis
    (E) none of the above

24. Which of the following characteristics of a drug can be measured by comparing the ED_{50}s for different responses to the same drug in vivo?

    (A) selectivity
    (B) specificity
    (C) therapeutic effectiveness
    (D) toxicity
    (E) reactivity

25. Which of the following strategies may be useful in mitigating the toxicity of a drug when the therapeutic and toxic effects are mediated by the same receptor?

    (A) administration of the drug at the lowest dose that produces acceptable benefit
    (B) manipulating the concentrations of the drug available in different parts of the body
    (C) utilization of adjunctive drugs that act through different receptor mechanisms to allow lowering of the dose of the first drug
    (D) all of the above
    (E) none of the above

26. What is the volume of distribution (V_d) of a drug whose concentration in the plasma is 1 µg/mL and the total amount of drug in the body is 42 mg?

    (A) 2.4 L
    (B) 4.2 L
    (C) 24 L
    (D) 42 L
    (E) 240 L

27. The rate of renal elimination of a drug in a 70-kg man is 10 mg/hr and the plasma concentration is 1 mg/L. What is the renal clearance of the drug?

    (A) 0.1 L/hr
    (B) 1.0 L/hr
    (C) 10 L/hr
    (D) 70 L/hr
    (E) 700 L/hr

28. Which of the following methods can be used to calculate the clearance of a drug when the rate of elimination is first order?

    (A) Clearance is the area under the curve (AUC) of the time-concentration profile after a dose.
    (B) Clearance is the AUC of the time-concentration profile after a dose divided by the dose.
    (C) Clearance is the dose divided by the AUC of the time-concentration profile after a dose.
    (D) Clearance is the dose multiplied by the AUC of the time-concentration profile after a dose.
    (E) none of the above

29. By what type of elimination is ethanol eliminated from the body?

    (A) first order
    (B) flow dependent
    (C) hyperbolic
    (D) pseudo-zero order
    (E) none of the above

30. What is the half-life of a drug that is eliminated by flow-dependent elimination and has a clearance of 7 L/hr and a volume of distribution of 100 liters?

    (A) 7 hours
    (B) 10 hours
    (C) 14 hours
    (D) 70 hours
    (E) 700 hours

31. If the dosing interval for a drug is one half-life and the peak plasma level after the first dose is 100 µg/mL, what will be the peak plasma level when a steady state is achieved?

    (A) 100 µg/mL
    (B) 200 µg/mL
    (C) 300 µg/mL
    (D) 400 µg/mL
    (E) 500 µg/mL

32. What is the extraction ratio for a drug if the hepatic clearance is 45 L/hr and the hepatic blood flow is 90 L/hr?

    (A) 0.1
    (B) 0.25
    (C) 0.5
    (D) 1.0
    (E) 2.0

33. What is the systemic bioavailability (F) of a drug whose extent of absorption (f) is 0.8 and extraction ratio (ER) is 0.3?

    (A) 0.24
    (B) 0.38
    (C) 0.56
    (D) 1.14
    (E) 2.67

34. Which of the following routes of administration avoid(s) the first-pass effect?

    (A) intramuscular
    (B) subcutaneous
    (C) sublingual
    (D) transdermal
    (E) all of the above

35. Suppose you want to give a drug by intravenous infusion at a dosing rate that would provide a target concentration of 20 mg/L. The clearance of the drug is 4 L/hr/70 kg. Which of the following would be the best dosing rate to use?

    (A) 20 mg/hr/70 kg
    (B) 40 mg/hr/70 kg
    (C) 60 mg/hr/70 kg
    (D) 80 mg/hr/70 kg
    (E) 100 mg/hr/70 kg

36. What would be the maintenance dose for administration of a drug every 12 hours if the calculated dosing rate were 40 mg/hr?

    (A) 120 mg
    (B) 240 mg
    (C) 480 mg
    (D) 960 mg
    (E) 1,920 mg

37. What would be the maintenance dose for oral administration of a drug every 8 hours if the calculated dosing rate were 20 mg/hr and the bioavailability were 0.5?

    (A) 40 mg
    (B) 75 mg
    (C) 110 mg
    (D) 240 mg
    (E) 320 mg

38. Assuming a one-compartment model, what would be the loading dose to achieve a target plasma concentration of 25 µg/L of a drug whose volume of distribution is 100 L?

    (A) 250 µg
    (B) 750 µg
    (C) 1,500 µg
    (D) 2,000 µg
    (E) 2,500 µg

39. Which of the following effects may result from the biotransformation of a drug by hepatic microsomal enzymes?

    (A) activation of a prodrug to a pharmacodynamically active compound
    (B) conversion of a lipophilic drug into a more water-soluble compound
    (C) conversion of a pharmacodynamically active drug into an inactive metabolite
    (D) all of the above
    (E) none of the above

40. Hepatic biotransformation reactions that unmask or introduce a functional group (OH, NH_2, or SH) are known as

   (A) conjugations
   (B) glucuronidations
   (C) phase I metabolism
   (D) phase II metabolism
   (E) synthetic reactions

41. Which of the following types of metabolic reactions are catalyzed by the microsomal mixed function oxidase system?

   (A) hydrolyses
   (B) oxidations
   (C) reductions
   (D) all of the above
   (E) none of the above

42. Cimetidine and ketoconazole are examples of drugs that

   (A) inactivate cytochrome P450 by irreversible binding to the heme iron
   (B) induce cytochrome P450 activity
   (C) induce microsomal transferases
   (D) inhibit cytochrome P450 by competitive inhibition
   (E) inhibit microsomal transferases by competitive inhibition

43. Which of the following is a phase II metabolic reaction?

   (A) acetylation
   (B) aliphatic hydroxylation
   (C) azo reduction
   (D) deamination
   (E) O-dealkylation

44. In which part of the cell are most cytochrome P450 enzymes located?

   (A) cell membrane
   (B) cytoplasm
   (C) nucleus
   (D) rough endoplasmic reticulum
   (E) smooth endoplasmic reticulum

45. Which of the following compounds is (are) known to induce cytochrome P450?

   (A) glucocorticoids
   (B) macrolide antibiotics
   (C) phenobarbital
   (D) polycyclic aromatic hydrocarbons
   (E) all of the above

46. CYP2B1 is an isozyme of what enzyme system?

   (A) cyclic nucleotide phosphodiesterase
   (B) epoxide hydrolase
   (C) mixed function oxidase
   (D) sulfotransferase
   (E) transmethylase

47. Which of the following is (are) nongenetic factors that account for individual variations in drug distribution, biotransformation, and elimination?

   (A) age
   (B) circadian rhythm
   (C) liver function
   (D) sex
   (E) all of the above

48. Which of the following dietary and environmental factors is (are) known to alter the rate of metabolism of drugs by the cytochrome P450 system?

   (A) charcoal-broiled foods
   (B) cigarette smoke
   (C) grapefruit juice
   (D) all of the above
   (E) none of the above

49. Which of the following drugs is (are) known to enhance the metabolism of other drugs by enzyme induction?

   (A) benzo[a]pyrene
   (B) phenobarbital
   (C) phenytoin
   (D) rifampin
   (E) all of the above

50. What is the main mechanism whereby rifampin alters the response to oral contraceptives?

    (A) It induces the enzymes that metabolize oral contraceptives to inactive products.
    (B) It inhibits ovulation by a direct effect on the ovaries.
    (C) It inhibits the enzymes that metabolize oral contraceptives to inactive products.
    (D) It interferes with the implantation of a fertilized ovum by a direct effect on the endometrium.
    (E) It interferes with the secretion of follicle-stimulating hormone (FSH) and luteinizing hormone (LH) by the pituitary gland.

51. In the search for new drugs, approximately how many new molecules must be synthesized for each new drug introduced?

    (A) 50 to 100
    (B) 200 to 400
    (C) 500 to 1,000
    (D) 2,000 to 4,000
    (E) 5,000 to 10,000

52. The development of the first useful H_2 histamine receptor antagonist, cimetidine, is an example of which kind of approach to drug discovery?

    (A) biotechnology and cloning of genes
    (B) chemical modification of a known molecule
    (C) random screening for biologic activity of large numbers of previously discovered chemical entities
    (D) rational drug design based on an understanding of biologic mechanisms and chemical structure
    (E) all of the above

53. The development of tissue plasminogen activator (t-PA) as a thrombolytic agent is an example of which kind of approach to drug discovery?

    (A) biotechnology and cloning of genes
    (B) chemical modification of a known molecule
    (C) random screening for biologic activity of large numbers of previously discovered chemical entities
    (D) rational drug design based on an understanding of biologic mechanisms and chemical structure
    (E) all of the above

DIRECTIONS (Questions 54 through 74): Each group of questions in this section consists of groups of lettered headings followed by lists of numbered words or phrases. For each numbered word or phrase, select the ONE lettered heading that is most closely associated with it. Each lettered heading may be selected once, more than once, or not at all.

Questions 54 through 57

Which phase of drug development is most closely associated with the characteristics in the numbered list?

    (A) animal testing
    (B) phase 1
    (C) phase 2
    (D) phase 3
    (E) phase 4

54. The effects of the drug as a function of dosage is usually studied in a small number (25 to 50) healthy volunteers.

55. Monitoring of the safety of the drug in a very large number of patients after the New Drug Application has been approved and the drug is marketed.

56. The drug is studied for the first time in patients with the target disease to determine its efficacy.

57. Initial evaluation of a new drug's toxicity is done in this phase.

Questions 58 through 64

Which legislation in the lettered headings is most closely associated with the descriptions in the following numbered list?

(A) Pure Food and Drug Act of 1906

(B) Opium Exclusion Act of 1909

(C) Amendment (1912) to the Pure Food and Drug Act

(D) Harrison Narcotic Act of 1914

(E) Food, Drug, and Cosmetic Act of 1938

(F) Durham–Humphrey Act of 1952

(G) Kefauver–Harris Amendments (1962) to the Food, Drug, and Cosmetic Act

(H) Comprehensive Drug Abuse Prevention and Control Act (1970)

(I) Orphan Drug Amendments of 1983

58. Provided incentives for development of drugs that treat diseases that occur in less than 200,000 patients in the United States

59. Required that all new drugs be safe

60. Required proof of efficacy for all new drugs

61. Prohibited mislabeling and adulteration of drugs

62. Gave the FDA power to determine which drugs can be sold without a prescription

63. Set controls on the manufacture of habit-forming drugs

64. This legislation was in part in response to the epidemic of birth defects caused by thalidomide

Questions 65 through 74

Which of the following mechanisms of action is most closely associated with the major pharmacological effects of each of the listed drugs?

(A) Activation of G proteins and second messengers

(B) Activation of ligand-regulated transmembrane enzymes including receptor tyrosine kinases

(C) Direct binding to and inhibition of an enzyme catalyzing a key metabolic reaction

(D) Opening or closing of ligand-gated ion channels

(E) Regulation of gene transcription by intracellular receptors

65. Gamma-aminobutyric acid (GABA)

66. Acetylcholine (acting on muscarinic receptors)

67. Acetylcholine (acting on nicotinic receptors)

68. Catecholamines (acting on $alpha_1$ adrenoceptors)

69. Catecholamines (acting on beta adrenoceptors)

70. Glucocorticoids

71. Insulin

72. Methotrexate

73. Thyroid hormones

74. Vitamin D

Answers and Explanations

1. **(E)** More than half of all useful drugs are chiral molecules. Different enantiomers of a drug are oriented differently around one or more asymmetric atoms within their molecular structures. This affects their ability to fit into receptor sites and active sites of enzymes. Therefore, different enantiomers of a drug commonly differ in the affinity of their binding to receptors, ability to activate receptors, and in the rate of their metabolism by drug-metabolizing enzymes. *(Katzung, p. 3).*

2. **(A)** Covalent bonds are the strongest of the bonds by which drugs may bind to their receptors. They are least likely to contribute to very selective drug action because weak bonds require a very precise fit of the drug to its receptor if an interaction is to occur, but covalent bonds do not require a precise fit. *(Katzung, pp. 2–3)*

3. **(B)** Antagonists bind to receptors but do not activate them, and therefore they do not produce any direct pharmacological effect. However, antagonists can block the effect of agonists and partial agonists by blocking access of the activating drugs to receptors. Agonists produce strong responses when they occupy their receptors, whereas partial agonists produce a weaker response with full receptor occupancy than agonists. Inverse agonists and inverse partial agonists produce effects opposite the effects produced by agonists and partial agonists. *(Katzung, pp. 11–16)*

4. **(B)** Lipid solubility is most important in the diffusion of drugs across lipid barriers or membranes that separate aqueous compartments of the body. Molecules that are insoluble in lipid may be transported by special carriers, endocytosis, or exocytosis. Solubility in water is most important for transport across aqueous compartments. *(Katzung, p. 5)*

5. **(C)** The formula for Fick's law is:

   Flux (molecules per unit time) =

   $$(C_1 - C_2) \times \frac{\text{Area} \times \text{Permeability coefficient}}{\text{Length of path}}$$

   C_1 is the higher concentration of the drug.
   C_2 is the lower concentration of the drug.
   Area is the area across which diffusion is occurring.
   Permeability coefficient is a measure of the mobility of the drug in the medium.
   Length of path is the length of the diffusion path of the drug. *(Katzung, p. 5)*

6. **(B)** The quaternary amine is bonded to four carbon atoms and therefore carries a permanent positive charge. Drug molecules that are primary, secondary, and tertiary amines carry an unshared pair of electrons and may undergo reversible protonation, thus varying their lipid solubility with pH. *(Katzung, p. 7)*

7. **(D)** Almost all drugs reach the urine by glomerular filtration. A significant fraction of lipid-soluble molecules will be reabsorbed as they pass down the renal tubule. Drugs that are weak acids or weak bases are lipid soluble in their un-ionized forms, but not in their ionized forms. A weak acid, such as aspirin, is ionized in its unprotonated form and, therefore, alkalinization of the urine using

sodium bicarbonate tends to trap the weak acid in the urine. A weak base is ionized in its protonated form and thus tends to be trapped in acidic urine. *(Katzung, pp. 5–7)*

8. **(C)** The ionization of a weak acid may be represented by HA $\leftrightarrow$ H$^+$ + A$^-$, whereas the ionization of a weak base may be represented by H$^+$ + B $\leftrightarrow$ HB$^+$. The degree of ionization of weak acids and weak bases can be calculated using the Henderson–Hasselbalch equation, which is:

log [(protonated)/(unprotonated)] = pK$_a$ – pH

The pK$_a$ is the pH at which the concentration of the ionized and un-ionized forms of the drug are equal. *(Katzung, pp. 5–6)*

9. **(D)** The ionization of a weak acid, such as theophylline, may be represented by HA $\leftrightarrow$ H$^+$ + A$^-$. Therefore, the un-ionized form of the drug is protonated and the ionized form is unprotonated. The Henderson–Hasselbalch equation is used to calculate the protonation, and therefore the ionization is:

log [(protonated)/(unprotonated)] = pK$_a$ – pH

In the problem presented, the log [(protonated)/(unprotonated)] = 8.8 – 7.8 = 1.0. Therefore, the ratio of (protonated)/(unprotonated) is 10/1. *(Katzung, pp. 5–6)*

10. **(D)** The avidity of the binding of a drug for a particular receptor depends on the size, shape, and electrical charge of the drug molecule. *(Katzung, p. 9)*

11. **(E)** The cardioactive digitalis glycosides are examples of drugs that produce their effects by interacting with transport proteins. Specifically, they inhibit Na$^+$/K$^+$ adenosine triphosphatase (ATPase) to produce their effects. Other proteins that serve as "receptors" for drugs are regulatory proteins, enzymes, and structural proteins. *(Katzung, pp. 9–11)*

12. **(A)** In the binding of a drug to its receptor, the higher the K$_D$ the lower the affinity, and the lower the K$_D$ the higher the affinity. Efficacy refers to how great the maximum effect

of a drug is as revealed by concentration-effect curves, and the EC$_{50}$ represents the drug concentration that produces 50% of the maximum effect. Intrinsic activity is a characteristic of the drug that is related to its efficiency in producing an effect when it occupies its targeted receptors. *(Katzung, pp. 11–14)*

13. **(A)** When plotted on linear axes, the relationship between the drug concentration and its effect is a hyperbolic curve. When the drug concentration is plotted on a logarithmic axis, the curve is sigmoidal in shape. These relationships are according to the following equation:

$$E = (E_{max} \times C) / (C + EC_{50})$$

E is the effect.
E$_{max}$ is the maximum effect produced by the drug.
C is the concentration of the drug.
EC$_{50}$ is the concentration of drug that produces 50% of E$_{max}$. *(Katzung, pp. 11–13)*

14. **(C)** The EC$_{50}$ of the agonist concentration-response curve will be increased by the competitive antagonist because the presence of the antagonist requires higher concentrations of agonist to produce the same effect. The maximum effect is not decreased because the binding of the competitive antagonist to the receptor is reversible and therefore can be surmounted by high concentrations of agonist. *(Katzung, pp. 14–15)*

15. **(E)** An irreversible antagonist will typically decrease the maximum effect of an agonist because it combines irreversibly with receptors, thereby effectively reducing the number of receptors available for the agonist to interact with. Since there are no "spare" receptors, the number of remaining receptors is inadequate for the agonist to produce the same maximum effect that it could in the absence of the irreversible antagonist. *(Katzung, pp. 14–15)*

16. **(B)** Protamine reverses the anticoagulant effects of heparin by binding to heparin mole-

cules and therefore is an example of a chemical antagonist. (*Katzung, p. 16*)

17. **(E)** Glucocorticoids can elevate blood sugar by their effects to increase glucose output from the liver and decrease glucose uptake by skeletal muscle. Insulin counteracts the elevated blood glucose by acting on a quite distinct receptor-effector system and therefore is an example of a physiological antagonist. (*Katzung, pp. 16–17*)

18. **(E)** In the continued presence of an agonist, the (beta-adrenoceptor is phosphorylated by beta-ARK (beta-adrenergic receptor kinase). A protein, beta-arrestin, binds to the phosphorylated receptor, blocking the receptor's activation of G_S. (*Katzung, p. 24*)

19. **(C)** The ED_{50} or EC_{50} of a drug describes the pharmacological potency of a drug. The potency often determines the dose that is prescribed. The efficacy of a drug reflects the upper limit of the response at high drug concentrations. (*Katzung, pp. 28–29*)

20. **(A)** Quantal dose-effect curves plot all-or-none types of responses in patient populations versus dose. The other choices in this question refer to graded responses. (*Katzung, pp. 28–30*)

21. **(E)** The therapeutic index is the ratio of the median toxic dose (TD_{50}) to the median effective dose (ED_{50}). The TD_{50} and ED_{50} are derived from quantal dose-effect plots. The larger the therapeutic index, the greater the margin of safety of the drug. (*Katzung, pp. 29–30*)

22. **(C)** An idiosyncratic drug response is one that occurs infrequently in patients. The other terms listed in this question all refer to quantitative variations in responsiveness. (*Katzung, p. 30*)

23. **(D)** Tachyphylaxis refers to a rapidly developing tolerance to a drug's effects. Idiosyncrasy refers to a drug response that occurs infrequently in patients. Hypersensitivity usually refers to an allergic or immunologic response. (*Katzung, p. 30*)

24. **(A)** Selectivity can be measured by comparing the ED_{50}s (median effective doses) for different effects of the drug in vivo. Specificity is an incorrect answer because drugs are generally not specific since they usually produce more than one effect. (*Katzung, p. 32*)

25. **(D)** All three of the therapeutic strategies that can be used to reduce the toxicity of a drug whose therapeutic and toxic effects are mediated by the same receptor are listed in this item. (*Katzung, p. 33*)

26. **(D)** The volume of distribution relates the amount of drug in the body to the concentration in the blood, plasma, or plasma water. The formula for calculation is V_d = Amount of drug in body / C. In the example given, C is the concentration in the plasma. Therefore, V_d = 42,000 μg / 1 μg per mL = 42,000 mL or 42 L, which is the approximate volume of body water in a 70-kg man. The V_d is an *apparent* volume and represents the volume that would contain the drug if it were *homogenously* distributed at the concentration in the blood, plasma, or plasma water. (*Katzung, pp. 35–36*)

27. **(C)** In its simplest form, the clearance (Cl) of a drug can be calculated as the rate of elimination divided by the concentration in the blood, plasma, or plasma water, depending on the concentration measured. Therefore, in this example, Cl = 10 mg per hour per 70 kg/1 mg per L = 10 L per hour per 70 kg. (*Katzung, p. 36*)

28. **(C)** If elimination is first order, the clearance can be calculated by dividing the dose by the AUC. (*Katzung, p. 40*)

29. **(D)** The process of pseudo-zero order elimination is commonly assumed for elimination of ethanol. Capacity-limited elimination of drugs follows the formula:

$$\text{Rate of elimination} = \frac{V_{max} \times C}{K_m + C}$$

C is the drug concentration and K_m is the concentration at which the rate of elimination is 50% of the V_{max}. At concentrations that are high relative to the K_m, the rate of elimination becomes nearly independent of the concentration or a pseudo-zero order process. *(Katzung, p. 40)*

30. **(B)** The formula for calculating the half-life is as follows:

$$t_{1/2} = \frac{0.7 \times V_d}{Cl}$$

V_d is the volume of distribution and Cl is the clearance. *(Katzung, pp. 40–41)*

31. **(B)** The peak concentration of a drug when it has reached steady state is the peak concentration achieved after the first dose multiplied by the accumulation factor. The accumulation factor can be calculated by the formula: Accumulation factor = 1 / (1 – Fraction remaining). The *fraction remaining* is the fraction of the drug remaining at the end of the dosing interval. In the example, the dosing interval was one half-life, so the fraction remaining at the end of the dosing interval was 0.5. Therefore, the accumulation factor = 1 / (1 – 0.5) = 1 / 0.5 = 2. The peak concentration at steady state would be 100 × 2 = 200. *(Katzung, p. 41)*

32. **(C)** The *extraction ratio* = hepatic clearance/hepatic blood flow. *(Katzung, pp. 42–43)*

33. **(C)** Bioavailability can be calculated according to the formula:

$$F = f \times (1 - ER)$$

F = systemic bioavailability
f = extent of absorption
ER = extraction ratio.
(Katzung, pp. 42–43)

34. **(E)** The first-pass effect refers to hepatic biotransformation of a drug that is absorbed into the hepatic portal system. All of the routes of administration listed in this item avoid transport of the drug by the hepatic portal system. *(Katzung, p. 43)*

35. **(D)** The dosing rate is calculated by the formula: Dosing rate = Clearance × Target concentration. In this example, Dosing rate = 4 L/hr/70 kg × 20 mg/L = 80 mg/hr/70 kg. *(Katzung, pp. 45–46)*

36. **(C)** The maintenance dose is calculated by the formula: Maintenance dose = Dosing rate × Dosing interval. In this example, Maintenance dose = 40 mg/hr × 12 hr. *(Katzung, pp. 45–46)*

37. **(E)** The oral maintenance dose is calculated by the formula: Oral maintenance dose = (Dosing rate / Bioavailability) × Dosing interval. In this example, Oral maintenance dose = (20 / 0.5) × 8 = 320. *(Katzung, pp. 45–46)*

38. **(E)** The loading dose is calculated by the formula: Loading dose = Volume of distribution × Target concentration. In this example, Loading dose = 100 × 25 = 2,500. *(Katzung, p. 46)*

39. **(D)** Biotransformation reactions in the body may produce metabolites that are pharmacodynamically more active, equivalent, or less active than the parent drug. Water solubility is usually increased. *(Katzung, p. 51)*

40. **(C)** Phase I reactions usually convert the parent drug to a more polar metabolite. They do this by introducing or unmasking a functional group ($-OH$, $-NH_2$, $-SH$). Glucuronidations are examples of phase II reactions, which are synthetic reactions and also known as conjugations. *(Katzung, p. 52)*

41. **(D)** Oxidations, reductions, and hydrolyses are all phase I reactions carried out by the microsomal mixed function oxidase system (cytochrome P450). *(Katzung, pp. 53–56)*

42. **(D)** Cimetidine and ketoconazole are examples of drugs that reduce the metabolism of

endogenous substrates or other coadministered drugs by cytochrome P450 as a result of competitive inhibition. *(Katzung, p. 56)*

43. **(A)** Acetylation is a synthetic or phase II reaction. The other reactions in this item are all phase I reactions. *(Katzung, pp. 53–59)*

44. **(E)** Most of the cytochrome P450 enzymes are associated with the smooth endoplasmic reticulum, which forms microsomes when the cells are homogenized and fractionated. *(Katzung, p. 53)*

45. **(E)** All of the compounds listed in this item are known inducers of cytochrome P450 and can increase the metabolism of coadministered drugs that are metabolized by the P450 system. *(Katzung, p. 55)*

46. **(C)** CYP2B1 is an isozyme of the microsomal mixed-function oxidase (cytochrome P450) system. It is one of the most studied isoforms and is induced by phenobarbital. *(Katzung, p. 56)*

47. **(E)** Nongenetic variables that account for individual pharmacokinetic differences among patients include age, sex, liver size, liver function, circadian rhythm, body temperature, nutrition, and environmental factors. *(Katzung, pp. 57–58)*

48. **(D)** Charbroiled foods can induce CYP4A enzymes. Cigarette smokers are known to metabolize some drugs more rapidly than nonsmokers because of enzyme induction. Grapefruit juice is known to inhibit CYP3A. *(Katzung, p. 60)*

49. **(E)** Many drugs are known to induce drug-metabolizing enzymes and they include all of the compounds listed in this item. As a result, dosages of coadministered drugs may need to be increased to compensate for the increased rate of metabolism. For example, the dose of warfarin may need to be increased if it is coadministered with rifampin. *(Katzung, pp. 60–61)*

50. **(A)** Rifampin interferes with the ability of oral contraceptives to prevent pregnancy by inducing the enzymes that metabolize oral contraceptives to inactive products. *(Katzung, pp. 60–61)*

51. **(E)** Part of the high cost of developing new drugs includes the labor invested in searching for new molecules that may lead to useful drugs. *(Katzung, p. 64)*

52. **(D)** The major approach used to develop cimetidine was rational drug design based on suspected existence of different histamine receptor subtypes. *(Katzung, pp. 64–65)*

53. **(A)** Diane Pennica and colleagues at Genentech determined the genetic code for an endogenous plasminogen activator and expressed the protein to produce recombinant tissue plasminogen activator. *(Katzung, pp. 66–67)*

54. **(B)** Phase 1 trials are done to establish the probable limits of the safe clinical dosage range of the new drug. Many predictable toxicities are detected in this phase. *(Katzung, p. 72)*

55. **(E)** Phase 4 involves monitoring the safety of the new drug under conditions of actual use after it is marketed. Important drug-induced effects having an incidence of 1:10,000 or less can be detected in phase 4. *(Katzung, p. 72)*

56. **(C)** Except in cases of very toxic drugs such as for treatment of cancer or AIDS, volunteers in phase 1 trials are normal, healthy subjects. Therefore, the first use of most drugs in patients who have the target disease is phase 2, with the goal of determining the efficacy of the drug for treatment of the disease. A single-blind design is often used. *(Katzung, p. 72)*

57. **(A)** In preclinical studies, acute, subacute, and chronic toxicities are often studied in animals. Acute toxicity studies evaluate the effects of large single doses of the drug up to the lethal level. Subacute and chronic toxicity

studies are important for drugs intended for chronic use in humans. *(Katzung, pp. 67–69)*

58. **(I)** The Orphan Drug Amendments of 1983 amended the Food, Drug, and Cosmetic Act of 1938 to provide incentives for treatment of diseases affecting fewer than 200,000 patients in the United States. The FDA maintains an office to provide special assistance and grants to investigators who wish to study these types of drugs. *(Katzung, pp. 71–73)*

59. **(E)** The Food, Drug, and Cosmetic Act of 1938 required that all drugs be safe as well as pure. Enforcement is by the FDA. *(Katzung, p. 71)*

60. **(G)** The Kefauver–Harris Amendments (1962) required proof of efficacy as well as safety for all new drugs and drugs released since 1938. *(Katzung, p. 71)*

61. **(A)** The Pure Food and Drug Act of 1906 was introduced partly in response to unsanitary and unethical practices in the meat-packing industry. *(Katzung, pp. 70–71)*

62. **(F)** The Durham–Humphrey Act of 1952 vested the FDA with the power to determine which drugs could be sold without a prescription. *(Katzung, p. 71)*

63. **(H)** The Comprehensive Drug Abuse Prevention and Control Act (1970) outlined controls for the manufacture, distribution, and prescribing of habit-forming drugs. *(Katzung, p. 71)*

64. **(G)** The Kefauver–Harris Amendments were stimulated in part by the increased incidence of a birth defect involving shortening or complete absence of the limbs that was shown to be related to the taking of thalidomide by pregnant mothers. *(Katzung, pp. 70–71)*

65. **(D)** The signaling mechanism associated with the major actions of GABA is activation of $GABA_A$ receptors, which opens chloride channels. *(Katzung, pp. 20–21)*

66. **(A)** Activation of muscarinic receptors by acetylcholine activates a G protein, G_q, which causes activation of the enzyme phospholipase C, resulting in increased levels of the second messenger IP_3 (inositol-1,4,5-triphosphate), which triggers the release of calcium from intracellular storage vesicles, and increased levels of diacylglycerol, which activates protein kinase C. *(Katzung, pp. 21–26)*

67. **(D)** Activation of nicotinic receptors by acetylcholine opens sodium channels, producing an excitatory postsynaptic potential. *(Katzung, pp. 20–21)*

68. **(A)** Activation of $alpha_1$ adrenoceptors by catecholamines activates the calcium-phosphoinositide signaling pathway. *(Katzung, p. 22)*

69. **(A)** Activation of beta adrenoceptors by catecholamines causes activation of a G protein, G_S, resulting in the activation of adenylyl cyclase, producing an increased rate of formation of the second messenger cyclic adenosine monophosphate (cAMP). *(Katzung, pp. 21–26)*

70. **(E)** Glucocorticoids are lipid-soluble compounds that diffuse across plasma membranes and bind to intracellular receptors. Their interaction with each protein receptor causes the dissociation of an hsp90 stabilizer and permits conversion of the receptor to an active configuration, which can bind target DNA sequences and regulate transcription. *(Katzung, pp. 18–20)*

71. **(B)** The insulin receptor has an extracellular hormone-binding domain and a cytoplasmic enzyme domain that contains a tyrosine kinase. Activation of the receptor causes activation of the tyrosine kinase, resulting in the phosphorylation of target proteins in the signaling pathway. *(Katzung, pp. 19–20)*

72. **(C)** The antineoplastic drug methotrexate binds to and inhibits the enzyme dihydrofolate reductase. *(Katzung, pp. 10–11)*

73. **(E)** Receptors for thyroid hormones stimulate the transcription of genes in the nucleus by binding to specific DNA sequences near the gene whose expression is to be regulated. *(Katzung, p. 18)*

74. **(E)** Receptors for vitamin D stimulate the transcription of genes in the nucleus by binding to specific DNA sequences near the gene whose expression is to be regulated. *(Katzung, p. 18)*

CHAPTER 2

Drugs Affecting the Autonomic Nervous System

Questions

DIRECTIONS (Questions 75 through 107): Each of the numbered items or incomplete statements in this section is followed by answers or by completions of the statement. Select the ONE lettered answer or completion that is BEST in each case.

75. You are treating a patient with bronchial asthma with an inhaled beta-adrenergic agonist. The patient calls your office complaining that the inhaler is not working. On questioning, it appears this person has an elevated heart rate. The most appropriate course of action is to

    (A) add an inhaled glucocorticoid to the regimen
    (B) administer a systemic glucocorticoid
    (C) immediately stop the use of the inhaled agonist
    (D) substitute an inhaled glucocorticoid for the beta-agonist
    (E) switch to a different inhaled agonist

76. The tachycardia associated with the use of alpha-adrenergic-blocking agents is most likely due to

    (A) blockade of the alpha$_2$-adrenergic receptors
    (B) elimination of beta-adrenergic receptor activity
    (C) inhibition of the cholinergic nervous innervation
    (D) reflex activation in a recumbent patient
    (E) the release of epinephrine from the adrenal gland

77. The most likely reason for selecting a beta-adrenergic agonist with intrinsic sympathomimetic activity is

    (A) agents without intrinsic sympathomimetic activity are subject to first pass metabolism
    (B) the need for an agent that has a prolonged duration of action
    (C) these types of agonists are very long acting due to the covalent bond they form with the receptor
    (D) the potential to have less depressant effect on the heart
    (E) to prevent reflex tachycardia

78. The use of beta-adrenergic agonists in bronchial asthma is mainly designed to

    (A) compete with alpha-adrenergic agonists
    (B) inhibit the airway inflammatory response
    (C) stimulate airway secretion
    (D) manage acute contraction of airway smooth muscle
    (E) prevent awakening during the night

79. A major clinically important advantage of noncatecholamines over catecholamines is

    (A) noncatecholamines have a lower potential to cause central nervous system stimulation
    (B) their duration of action is longer
    (C) they are more effective in treating acute allergic reactions
    (D) they are not naturally occurring
    (E) they have a structure that permits parenteral administration

80. The effectiveness of beta-adrenergic blocking agents in treating essential hypertension is most likely due to

    (A) a combination of inhibition of cardiac output and renin release
    (B) inhibition of calcium entry into blood vessels
    (C) stimulation of vagal nerves, leading to increased circulating levels of acetylcholine
    (D) the direct blockade of angiotensin receptors
    (E) the production of nitric oxide

81. Low concentrations of which of the following agents administered on a background of low adrenergic nervous system activation can be expected to increase blood flow to the kidney?

    (A) cocaine
    (B) dopamine
    (C) epinephrine
    (D) phenylephrine
    (E) tyramine

82. Which of the following agents causes increased peripheral resistance due to the inhibition of reuptake at noradrenergic synapses?

    (A) cocaine
    (B) dopamine
    (C) epinephrine
    (D) phenylephrine
    (E) tyramine

83. Administration of which of the following will lead to an increase in peripheral resistance without cardiac stimulation?

    (A) cocaine
    (B) dopamine
    (C) epinephrine
    (D) phenylephrine
    (E) tyramine

84. Alpha-adrenergic blocking agents will convert which of the following vasoconstrictors to a vasodilator?

    (A) cocaine
    (B) dopamine
    (C) epinephrine
    (D) phenylephrine
    (E) tyramine

85. When it is desirable to administer an agent that will lower peripheral resistance but does not cause an increase in catecholamine release from the adrenergic nerve ending, prazosin is selected as the agent. Its mechanism of action is

    (A) activation of $beta_1$ receptors
    (B) elimination of the effects of $beta_2$ receptor activation
    (C) nonequilibrium alpha-adrenergic receptor blockade
    (D) selective blockade of $alpha_1$ receptors
    (E) specific activation of $alpha_2$ receptors

86. In choosing a noncatecholamine versus a catecholamine, which of the following factors is important?

    (A) Noncatecholamines have a shorter duration of action.
    (B) Catecholamines are effective only if administered orally.
    (C) Noncatecholamines are metabolized at a more rapid rate.

(D) Catecholamines are considered indirect-acting agents since they must enter the nerve ending and release norepinephrine.

(E) Noncatecholamines tend to have greater action on the central nervous system (CNS).

87. The administration of an adrenergic amine to a patient taking a tricyclic antidepressant may result in an unexpected elevation of blood pressure. The mechanism responsible for this effect is most likely

(A) increased sensitivity of the tissue to norepinephrine

(B) increased activity of catechol-O-methyl-transferase (COMT)

(C) interference with uptake of the amine into adrenergic nerve endings

(D) increased activity of monoamine oxidase (MAO)

(E) decreased destruction of the amine by metabolic enzymes

88. Increasing cardiac output with a selective $beta_1$-adrenergic agonist causes less tachycardia than increasing cardiac output with a nonselective beta agonist because

(A) the vasodilator action at $beta_2$ receptors is absent

(B) $beta_1$-receptor agonists cause upregulation of receptors

(C) nonselective agents are less potent

(D) selective agents are very specific for the heart and do not block other sites

(E) alpha receptors are inactivated by $beta_1$ selective agents

89. Which of the following is an accepted therapeutic use of epinephrine?

(A) treatment of pheochromocytoma

(B) combination with local anesthetics in 1:10,000 concentrations

(C) intravenous (IV) infusion for hemorrhagic shock

(D) treatment of acute hypersensitivity reaction to drugs

(E) cardiogenic shock

90. In the treatment of glaucoma, timolol would be preferred over propranolol because

(A) propranolol has a longer duration of action

(B) propranolol is nonselective

(C) propranolol will depress the heart

(D) timolol does not have local anesthetic activity

(E) timolol has intrinsic sympathomimetic activity

91. A gardener has been concerned about insects eating the vegetables he worked diligently to cultivate. He decides to use an insecticide to prevent any damage to his crop. His wife finds him in the gardening shed with signs of intoxication. Cholinesterase inhibitors

(A) cannot be reactivated until the enzyme inhibitor has "aged"

(B) do not affect skeletal muscle nicotinic receptors

(C) like edrophonium have duration of action lasting hours

(D) of the neostigmine type are effective in reversing the central effects of atropine intoxication

(E) are used to treat myasthenia gravis and may cause excessive salivation

92. The vasodilator activity of acetylcholine is due to

(A) an influx of calcium ion following calcium channel activation

(B) blockade of the release of norepinephrine

(C) release of endothelial relaxing factor (EDRF)

(D) stimulation of muscarinic receptors

(E) stimulation of nicotinic receptor

93. Studies conducted on patients who have survived myocardial infarctions show a reduction in mortality if they are maintained on

    (A) dobutamine
    (B) metaproterenol
    (C) nitroglycerin
    (D) phentolamine
    (E) timolol

94. In the treatment of diseases of the eye, which of the following choices would be appropriate?

    (A) placing eyedrops containing pilocarpine to relax the ciliary muscle
    (B) the administration of an adrenergic amine to produce mydriasis and cycloplegia
    (C) the use of diuretics to stimulate the kidney and reduce systemic fluids
    (D) the use of beta-adrenergic blocking agents to reduce the formation of aqueous humor in glaucoma

95. Activation of which of the following results in inhibition of cardiac muscle contraction?

    (A) alpha$_1$ receptors
    (B) beta$_1$ receptors
    (C) beta$_2$ receptors
    (D) dopamine D$_1$ receptors
    (E) muscarinic M$_2$ receptors

96. Activation of which of the following results in contraction of vascular smooth muscle?

    (A) alpha$_1$ receptors
    (B) beta$_1$ receptors
    (C) beta$_2$ receptors
    (D) dopamine D$_1$ receptors
    (E) muscarinic M$_2$ receptors

97. Which of the following neuromuscular blocking agents has the most rapid onset of action?

    (A) atracurium
    (B) metocurine
    (C) pancuronium
    (D) rapacuronium
    (E) tubocurarine

98. Which of the following neuromuscular blocking agents has the shortest duration of action when a single dose is administered?

    (A) pancuronium
    (B) pipecuronium
    (C) rocuronium
    (D) succinylcholine
    (E) vecuronium

99. Which of the following neuromuscular-blocking agents is broken down spontaneously in the body to form laudanosine and a related quaternary acid?

    (A) atracurium
    (B) metocurine
    (C) pancuronium
    (D) rapacuronium
    (E) tubocurarine

100. Which of the following is the most accurate description of tubocurarine?

    (A) ganglionic-blocking agent
    (B) muscarinic agonist
    (C) nicotinic agonist
    (D) noncompetitive neuromuscular-blocking agent
    (E) nondepolarizing neuromuscular-blocking agent

101. Which of the following drugs is accurately classified as a depolarization type of neuromuscular blocking agent?

    (A) atracurium
    (B) metocurine
    (C) succinylcholine
    (D) tubocurarine
    (E) vecuronium

102. Which of the following terms most accurately characterizes the phase II neuromuscular blockade produced by succinylcholine?

    (A) depolarizing block
    (B) desensitizing block
    (C) flexible block

(D) rigid block

(E) tetanus-producing block

103. Which of the following types of neuromuscular blockade respond(s) to tetanus-producing nerve stimulations by manifesting a diminished, but constant amplitude of contractile responses?

(A) nondepolarizing blockade

(B) phase I depolarizing blockade

(C) phase II depolarizing blockade

(D) all of the above

(E) none of the above

104. Which of the following neuromuscular blocking agents produces transient muscle fasciculations during its onset of action?

(A) atracurium

(B) rapacuronium

(C) succinylcholine

(D) tubocurarine

(E) vecuronium

105. Which of the following neuromuscular blocking agents produces a moderate block of cardiac muscarinic receptors, but no effect on autonomic ganglia and no tendency to cause release of histamine?

(A) atracurium

(B) metocurine

(C) pancuronium

(D) succinylcholine

(E) tubocurarine

106. Which of the following drugs produces the most pronounced cardiovascular effects?

(A) pipecuronium

(B) rapacuronium

(C) rocuronium

(D) tubocurarine

(E) vecuronium

107. Which of the following drugs produces a neuromuscular blockade that is least likely to be reversed by neostigmine?

(A) atracurium

(B) metocurine

(C) succinylcholine

(D) tubocurarine

(E) vecuronium

DIRECTIONS (Questions 108 through 156): Each group of questions in this section consists of groups of lettered headings followed by lists of numbered words or phrases. For each numbered word or phrase, select the ONE lettered heading that is most closely associated with it. Each lettered heading may be selected once, more than once, or not at all.

Questions 108 through 110

Beta-adrenergic blocking agents can be utilized based on several properties listed below. For each condition listed, select the proper choice of an agent.

(A) cardioselectivity

(B) beta$_2$ selectivity

(C) duration of action

(D) intrinsic sympathomimetic activity

(E) nonequilibrium blockade

108. There is concern about a patient who may forget to take a dose of the drug due to memory impairment.

109. A patient with a history of bronchial asthma develops atrial arrhythmias, and it is deemed appropriate to place the individual on a beta-adrenergic blocking agent.

110. In the operating room, a patient develops an arrhythmia and the choice of esmolol as the most desirable agent is most likely based on _____.

Questions 111 through 114

Match the appropriate drug to its action.

    (A) butoxamine

    (B) carvedilol

    (C) phenoxybenzamine

    (D) prazosin

    (E) salmeterol

    (F) tramsulosin

111. Selective action on the $alpha_{1A}$-adrenergic receptor

112. Blocks $beta_2$-adrenergic receptors

113. Used in hypertension and congestive heart failure because it decreases peripheral resistance and protects the heart from abnormal cardiac rhythms

114. Forms ethyleneimonium ions

Questions 115 through 120

Match the result of activation of the following receptors with a physiologic response.

    (A) $alpha_1$

    (B) $alpha_2$

    (C) $beta_1$

    (D) $beta_2$

    (E) muscarinic

    (F) nicotinic

115. Bradycardia

116. Bronchodilation

117. Vasoconstriction

118. Dilation of skeletal muscle vascular beds

119. Release of adrenal catecholamines

120. Inhibition of norepinephrine release

Questions 121 through 123

Match the appropriate drug with its use.

    (A) acetylcholine

    (B) carbachol

    (C) bethanechol

    (D) methacholine

    (E) choline

121. Predominantly used for its cardiovascular effects

122. Primarily used to increase tone of the urinary retention and not hydrolyzed by cholinesterases

123. Not employed therapeutically because of its rapid hydrolysis and lack of specificity

Questions 124 through 126

Match the appropriate agent with each statement below.

    (A) muscarinic agonists

    (B) anticholinergic agents

    (C) ganglionic-blocking drugs

    (D) nicotinic agonists

    (E) nicotinic antagonists

124. Contraindications include asthma, coronary insufficiency, and peptic ulcer.

125. Signs of toxicity may include hot, dry skin and delirium.

126. Stimulates both skeletal muscle and ganglionic sites.

Questions 127 through 130

Match the appropriate agent with the actions below.

    (A) atropine

    (B) botulinum toxin

    (C) hemicholinium

    (D) synaptobrevin

    (E) vesamicol

127. Inhibits the release of acetylcholine from cholinergic fibers

128. A cellular protein that promotes fusion of the vesicular membrane

129. Alters the storage of acetylcholine in dense core vesicles

130. Blocks the reuptake of choline into cholinergic fibers

Questions 131 through 134

Match the appropriate agent with its action below.

    (A) bretylium
    (B) glucocorticoids
    (C) metyrosine
    (D) reserpine
    (E) tricyclic antidepressants

131. Inhibits the rate-limiting enzyme responsible for norepinephrine synthesis

132. Inhibits the uptake of norepinephrine into extraneuronal sites

133. Leads to loss of granular storage of norepinephrine

134. Inhibits norepinephrine release from adrenergic nerve endings

Questions 135 through 138

Match the appropriate enzyme with the correct statement below.

    (A) COMT
    (B) dopamine beta hydroxylase
    (C) MAO
    (D) phenylethanolamine N-methyltransferase (PNMT)
    (E) thyroid hormone (TH)

135. Found in the effluent following adrenergic nerve stimulation

136. Inhibition leads to dangerous increases in blood pressure when fermented foods are ingested

137. Responsible for synthesis of epinephrine

138. Leads to the production of normetanephrine

Questions 139 through 142

In all of the traces provided, assume that blood pressure was recorded from the carotid artery and drugs administered through an indwelling catheter in the femoral vein. Animals were anesthetized with 30 mg/kg of pentobarbital sodium. (See Fig. 2.1 on page 24.)

    (A) atropine
    (B) neostigmine
    (C) phentolamine
    (D) pralidoxime
    (E) propranolol

139. Drug A

140. Drug B

141. Drug C

142. Drug D

Questions 143 through 146 (See Fig. 2.2 on page 24)

    (A) epinephrine
    (B) isoproterenol
    (C) metaproterenol
    (D) norepinephrine
    (E) phenylephrine

143. Drug A

144. Drug B

145. Drug C

146. Drug D

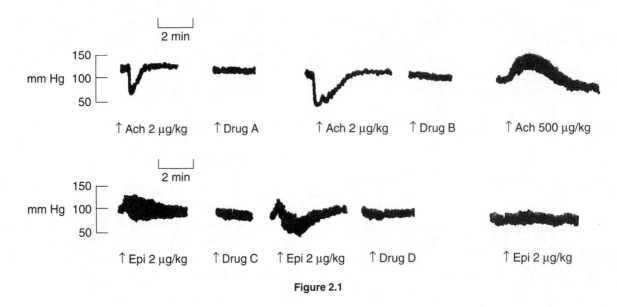

Figure 2.1

Questions 147 through 150

Using Figure 2.3 on page 25, answer the following questions. The letters in the diagram refer to processes occurring in the adrenergic nerve ending.

147. Bretylium inhibits this process.

148. Activation of this site will result in effector activation.

149. Indirect-acting amines release norepinephrine from this site.

150. Stimulation of this site will inhibit norepinephrine release.

Questions 151 through 156

Match the reaction with the appropriate receptor.

(A) alpha$_1$ receptors

(B) alpha$_2$ receptors

(C) beta$_1$ receptors

(D) beta$_2$ receptors

(E) beta$_3$ receptors

(F) dopamine D$_1$ receptors

(G) dopamine D$_2$ receptors

(H) dopamine D$_3$ receptors

(I) muscarinic M$_1$ receptors

(J) muscarinic M$_2$ receptors

(K) nicotinic N$_M$ receptors

(L) nicotinic N$_N$ receptors

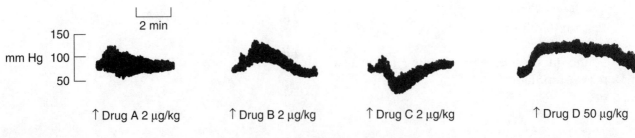

Figure 2.2

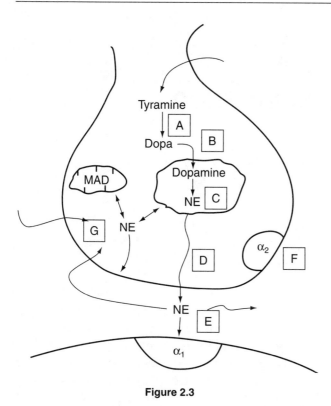

Figure 2.3

151. Skeletal muscle contraction

152. Activation of the phosphoinositide pathway in CNS neurons and sympathetic postganglionic neurons

153. Renal vasodilation

154. Smooth muscle relaxation

155. Ganglionic stimulation

156. Primary location is on lipocytes

Answers and Explanations

75. (C) The administration of inhaled glucocorticoids is for maintenance therapy, and simply adding this agent may cause upregulation of beta receptors, worsening the situation. The use of systemic glucocorticoids is reserved for management of airway reactivity, and the problem here appears to be the accelerated heart rate. Substituting an inhaled glucocorticoid for the beta agonist may be useful but probably not the most immediate course of action. Adding a different inhaled agonist would not be expected to improve the problem of receptor downregulation. Even though this point is arguable, the cautious approach is to discontinue the agonist. *(Katzung, pp. 341, 343)*

76. (A) The most obvious answer is the inhibition of alpha$_2$-shutdown of norepinephrine release. Neither beta receptors nor muscarinic receptors are altered, and epinephrine release would be expected only in someone who is standing. Standing reflexes are not present in a recumbent patient. *(Katzung, pp. 139–140)*

77. (D) Since compounds of this type have partial agonist activity, they depress the heart less (beta$_2$ > beta$_1$ activity). The metabolism, duration of action, and covalent bonding are not relevant issues. These agents would not be any more effective in preventing reflex tachycardia than any other beta blockers. *(Katzung, pp. 148, 167)*

78. (D) Beta-adrenergic agonists are used to relax airway smooth muscle acutely by increasing cyclic adenosine monophosphate (cAMP) levels. This is a beta$_2$-adrenergic receptor effect. *(Katzung, p. 129)*

79. (B) The major reason for selecting these agents is that they have oral effectiveness, are longer acting, or penetrate into the CNS. Some of them (e.g., ephedrine) are naturally occurring; they are less effective than catecholamines in treating acute allergic reactions, and their structure does not offer a solubility advantage. *(Katzung, pp. 130–131)*

80. (A) The major reasons beta-adrenergic blocking agents lower blood pressure are due to these two effects. These agents are not classes of calcium channel blockers, vagal nerve stimulants, or activators of nitric oxide. *(Katzung, p. 145)*

81. (B) At low doses the activation of D$_1$ receptors in the renal beds may lead to vasodilation and increased blood flow. As the dose of dopamine increases, beta$_1$-adrenergic receptors in the heart are activated. With even higher doses, alpha$_1$-adrenergic receptors in the skin vascular beds are activated leading to a progressive increase in peripheral resistance. *(Katzung, p. 130)*

82. (A) Cocaine, a local anesthetic, blocks the reuptake of norepinephrine, which results in a major increase in peripheral resistance. In the CNS, cocaine inhibits the reuptake of dopamine, leading to sensations that are intensely pleasurable. *(Katzung, p. 131)*

83. (D) Phenylephrine is one of a group of drugs that will cause an increase in peripheral resistance due to its selective activation of alpha$_1$-adrenergic receptors in skin vascular beds. *(Katzung, pp. 122, 130)*

84. **(C)** This is the classic "epinephrine reversal response." Because epinephrine nonselectively activates both alpha- (alpha$_1$ and alpha$_2$) and beta- (beta$_1$ and beta$_2$) adrenergic receptors, the response following alpha blockade (vasoconstriction) results in beta$_2$ receptor-induced vasodilation due to relaxation of blood vessels in skeletal muscle vascular beds. *(Katzung, pp. 122, 140)*

85. **(D)** Prazosin is an antihypertensive agent that reduces blood pressure by selectively blocking receptors on blood vessels. This results in a decrease in peripheral resistance. Even though tachycardia may occur due to reflex effects, there is no blockade of the process that inhibits norepinephrine release from adrenergic nerve endings. *(Katzung, p. 141)*

86. **(E)** Noncatecholamines are resistant to enzymatic inactivation by MAO and COMT. This fact means they have a longer duration of action, are orally effective, and are indirect acting (release norepinephrine from the adrenergic nerve ending). These compounds (e.g., dextroamphetamine) tend to penetrate to the CNS. *(Katzung, pp. 120, 130)*

87. **(C)** Tricyclic antidepressants along with cocaine block the transport system in the axonal membrane of the adrenergic nerve terminal. This is the major pathway for termination of the response, and inhibiting this process results in a greater amount of the adrenergic amine in the vicinity of the receptor. *(Katzung, p. 80)*

88. **(A)** Nonselective agents will activate beta$_2$ receptors in skeletal muscle vascular beds, leading to a reflex tachycardia. Isoproterenol (nonselective) causes greater increases in heart rate than does dobutamine (selective). *(Katzung, p. 131)*

89. **(D)** Epinephrine, 1:1,000, is a time-honored drug used to treat acute hypersensitivity reactions to drugs and other allergens. It is also widely used with local anesthetics to delay absorption and prolong anesthesia; however, concentrations of 1:200,000 to 1:100,000 are employed for this purpose. *(Katzung, pp. 133–134)*

90. **(D)** When treating glaucoma, it is important that local anesthesia does not occur since lack of sensation in the eye could easily result in damage to the cornea. Timolol does not have intrinsic sympathomimetic activity, local anesthetic activity, or selectivity. Its duration of action is standard, approximately 4 hours. *(Katzung, pp. 145–147)*

91. **(E)** Myasthenia gravis is often treated with cholinesterase inhibitors, such as neostigmine, that do not cross the blood–brain barrier. Edrophonium, a short-acting agent, is useful in diagnosing myasthenia gravis. These agents cause signs of excessive muscarinic receptor activation, including excessive salivation. Atropine will antagonize these effects without suppressing the effect on nicotinic skeletal muscle sites. *(Katzung, p. 103)*

92. **(C)** The most correct answer is the release of EDRF (nitric oxide). A Nobel prize was awarded for the discovery that intact (in vivo) blood vessels released nitric oxide, which increased cyclic guanosine monophosphate and thus caused relaxation of blood vessels. Vessels with the endothelium removed contract in response to acetylcholine. *(Katzung, p. 97)*

93. **(E)** The Norwegian multicenter study of timolol after acute myocardial infarction demonstrated a reduction in mortality with 6-year follow-up. Propranolol and metoprolol also prolong survival. *(Katzung, p. 149)*

94. **(D)** Timolol is a beta-adrenergic blocking agent that reduces the secretion of aqueous humor from the ciliary epithelium. *(Katzung, pp. 150–151)*

95. **(E)** The activation of cardiac muscarinic M_2 receptors results in opening of potassium channels, and inhibition of adenylyl cyclase leading to a decrease in contractile force development. *(Katzung, pp. 83–85)*

96. **(A)** The major control of peripheral resistance is through activation of alpha$_1$-adrenergic receptors. This is a consequence of acti-vation of the phosphoinositide cascade and increased levels of IP$_3$ levels. *(Katzung, pp. 83–85)*

97. **(D)** Rapacuronium has the most rapid onset of action of the nondepolarizing neuromuscular blocking agents, and it has a duration of action of about 10 to 20 minutes. It is useful for procedures requiring a rapid induction of neuromuscular blockade and a short duration of action such as endotracheal intubation. *(Katzung, pp. 450–451)*

98. **(D)** Succinylcholine has a relatively brief duration of action of less than 8 minutes mainly due to its rapid hydrolysis by plasma cholinesterase. *(Katzung, pp. 450–451)*

99. **(A)** Laudanosine has little or no neuromuscular-blocking activity, but it has a relatively long elimination half-life and can cause seizures if it reaches high concentrations in the blood. *(Katzung, pp. 450–451)*

100. **(E)** Tubocurarine blocks the neuromuscular junction by surmountable blockade of postjunctional nicotinic receptors. *(Katzung, p. 451)*

101. **(C)** Succinylcholine is the only depolarizing neuromuscular-blocking agent presently in use in the United States. It blocks the neuromuscular junction by combining with nicotinic receptors to cause depolarization of the motor end plate and adjacent membranes. *(Katzung, pp. 451–452)*

102. **(B)** After prolonged exposure to succinylcholine, the postjunctional membrane becomes repolarized, but it is resistant to depolarization by acetylcholine. The exact mechanism for this desensitizing blockade is unclear. *(Katzung, p. 452)*

103. **(B)** Whereas the amplitude of the contractile responses to a tetanus-producing train of nerve stimuli is constant with a phase I depolarizing blockade, it fades with time with phase II depolarizing blockade and nondepolarizing blockade. *(Katzung, p. 453)*

104. **(C)** The transient muscle fasciculations, which are most prominent over the chest and abdomen, are probably associated with the depolarization caused by succinylcholine during its onset of action. *(Katzung, p. 454)*

105. **(C)** Pancuronium produces a moderate blockade of cardiac muscarinic receptors, which is the main mechanism responsible for the moderate increase in heart rate caused by this drug. *(Katzung, p. 455)*

106. **(D)** Tubocurarine produces hypotension, which is principally caused by its release of histamine and, in larger doses, to its ganglionic-blocking action. *(Katzung, p. 455)*

107. **(C)** The neuromuscular blockade produced by nondepolarizing agents is reversed by neostigmine and other cholinesterase inhibitors because the accumulation of acetylcholine at the neuromuscular junction tends to reverse the surmountable blockade produced by the nondepolarizing agents. Accumulation of acetylcholine at the neuromuscular junction does not reverse the phase I depolarizing blockade produced by succinylcholine. In addition, neostigmine inhibits the enzyme (plasma cholinesterase) responsible for the inactivation of succinylcholine. *(Katzung, p. 457)*

108. **(D)** The agents that have intrinsic sympathomimetic activity (ISA) or partial agonist activity (PAA) are characterized as preferred agents in this case since they may be less prone to cause rebound hypertension if a patient misses a dose of the drug. The overall clinical significance of this effect is unclear. *(Katzung, p. 148)*

109. **(A)** Beta-adrenergic blocking agents that are selective for the heart (beta$_1$) would be preferred. These types of agents, when used in the lower dosage range, have selective actions on the heart without adversely affecting airway smooth muscle. This property would be particularly important in patients with asthma. *(Katzung, pp. 146–147)*

110. **(C)** Esmolol can be administered intravenously in the operating room to suppress arrhythmias. It has a short (10 min) duration of action, making it a relatively safe agent for reversing the arrhythmia. The short duration of action is due to the fact that it is an ester that is rapidly hydrolyzed by plasma esterases. *(Katzung, p. 148)*

111. **(F)** Tramsulosin is a competitive alpha$_1$ blocking agent with selectivity for alpha$_{1A}$ receptors over alpha$_{1B}$ receptors. The efficacy of tramsulosin in benign prostatic hypertrophy (BPH) suggests that the alpha$_{1A}$ receptor is important in mediating prostate smooth-muscle contraction. *(Katzung, p. 141)*

112. **(A)** There is currently no clinical use for butoxamine, but it is employed in experimental studies to define receptor types. *(Katzung, p. 148)*

113. **(B)** Carvedilol is a nonselective beta-adrenergic blocking agent with alpha$_1$ selective blocking activity. Thus, this agent would protect the heart from catecholamine-induced arrhythmias and lower peripheral resistance to effectively increase cardiac output while reducing the energy required. The drug also appears to inhibit mitogenesis of vascular smooth muscle. *(Katzung, p. 148)*

114. **(C)** Phenoxybenzamine, a nonequilibrium alpha-adrenergic blocking agent, forms an ethyleneimonium ion when placed in solution. This occurs as a result of the ethylene side chain "cyclizing" with the nitrogen. The charge exists on the nitrogen but transfers to the carbon, making a highly reactive carbonium ion. This ion has a short half-life and it binds covalently to the receptor, effectively permanently removing the receptor's function. These agents are modeled after the nitrogen mustards (war gases). *(Katzung, p. 138)*

115. **(E)** Stimulation of muscarinic receptors in the heart will lead to slowing of the heart rate. These are M$_2$ receptors, which act by opening potassium channels and inhibiting adenylyl cyclase. *(Katzung, p. 83)*

116. **(D)** Airway smooth muscle relaxes when beta$_2$-adrenergic receptors are stimulated. This receptor activation results from stimulating adenylyl cyclase, resulting in an increase in cAMP. *(Katzung, pp. 124, 127)*

117. **(A)** The predominance of alpha$_1$ receptors on vascular smooth muscle in skin beds leads to an increase in peripheral resistance when these receptors are stimulated. *(Katzung, p. 127)*

118. **(D)** Activation of beta$_2$ receptors in skeletal muscle vascular beds delivers increased blood flow to these tissues. *(Katzung, pp. 123–124)*

119. **(F)** Catecholamine release from the adrenal gland is mediated by nicotinic receptors. The adrenal gland is similar to a large ganglion, and stimulation results in an increase in circulating epinephrine. *(Katzung, p. 92)*

120. **(B)** Vascular smooth muscle contains alpha$_2$ receptors, which, when stimulated, provide a negative feedback on norepinephrine release from adrenergic nerve endings. *(Katzung, pp. 80, 126, 127)*

121. **(D)** Methacholine has selectivity for muscarinic versus nicotinic receptors and is hydrolyzed at a slower rate by acetylcholine esterase than acetylcholine. It is resistant to nonspecific cholinesterase. *(Katzung, pp. 94–95)*

122. **(C)** The primary action of bethanechol is to increase urinary bladder tone and to increase tone of the lower esophageal sphincter in patients with reflux esophagitis. It is not hydrolyzed by cholinesterases. *(Katzung, pp. 95, 103)*

123. **(A)** Because acetylcholine is so rapidly hydrolyzed, it has virtually no therapeutic use. Derivatives that have resistance to enzymatic degradation have been synthesized to provide longer duration of action and some selectivity at organ sites. *(Katzung, pp. 79, 95)*

124. **(A)** Agents that activate the muscarinic receptor may produce untoward effects in patients with underlying conditions. In asthmatics they cause bronchial smooth-muscle contraction. In patients with angina pectoris, the danger is a hypotensive response that may reduce coronary blood flow. In patients with gastric ulcer, the stimulation of gastric acid secretion would be undesirable. *(Katzung, p. 96)*

125. **(B)** Intoxication with atropine or plants containing anticholinergic agents may include a rapid/weak pulse, flushed skin (scarlet color), widely dilated pupils, and ataxia. The old adage is used to describe anticholinergic intoxication: dry as a bone, blind as a bat, red as a beet, and mad as a hatter. This alkaloid produces both peripheral cholinergic blockade and central nervous system effects. *(Katzung, p. 116)*

126. **(D)** Ganglionic stimulants such as nicotine do not show specificity for nicotine receptors. The effects observed are unpredictable, since nicotine has low selectivity at nicotinic sites and it first stimulates then blocks receptors. The major interest in nicotine is related to its acute and chronic toxicity. However, the use of nicotine patches has led to a renewed interest in this compound in other disease states. *(Katzung, p. 104)*

127. **(B)** Botulinum toxin inhibits vesicular release of acetylcholine by enzymatic removal of two amino acids from fusion proteins. *(Katzung, p. 79)*

128. **(D)** Calcium ion destabilizes the acetylcholine-containing vesicles by interacting with vesicular membrane association proteins (synaptotagmin and synaptobrevin)

and terminal membrane proteins (SNAP-25). *(Katzung, p. 79)*

129. **(E)** The antiporter that removes protons and allows storage of acetylcholine in the vesicles can be inhibited by vesamicol. *(Katzung, p. 78)*

130. **(C)** A group of compounds called hemicholiniums block a sodium-dependent membrane carrier, which recovers the choline from hydrolyzed acetylcholine. *(Katzung, p. 78)*

131. **(C)** The tyrosine analog metyrosine inhibits tyrosine hydroxylase, the rate-limiting enzyme in norepinephrine biosynthesis. *(Katzung, p. 81)*

132. **(B)** Extraneuronal uptake, referred to as uptake$_2$, is inhibited by glucocorticoids. These agents also stimulate the synthesis of epinephrine in the adrenal gland. *(Katzung, pp. 81–82)*

133. **(D)** The high-affinity carrier for catecholamines, which is responsible for concentrating catecholamines in the storage granule, is inhibited by reserpine alkaloids. These agents deplete several biogenic amines both in the periphery and in the CNS. *(Katzung, pp. 80–81)*

134. **(A)** Bretylium is a local anesthetic sodium channel blocker that concentrates in adrenergic nerve endings and paralyzes the release mechanism for norepinephrine. *(Katzung, p. 80)*

135. **(B)** When dopamine enters the granular vesicle, its beta carbon is hydroxylated to norepinephrine. With nerve stimulation, the contents of the granule, including dopamine hydroxylase, are released. *(Katzung, p. 81)*

136. **(C)** Ingestion of indirect-acting amines found in fermented foods (beer, cheese, wine) can result in the release of large amounts of norepinephrine that has accumulated in adrenergic nerve endings when monoamine oxidase inhibitors (MAOIs) are administered as antidepressants. *(Katzung, p. 505)*

137. **(D)** In the adrenal gland, norepinephrine is converted to epinephrine by the addition of a methyl group on the nitrogen. This process is catalyzed by PNMT. *(Katzung, p. 81)*

138. **(A)** COMT O-methylates the hydroxy group on the ring structure of catecholamines, thus rendering them inactive. Norepinephrine is converted to normetanephrine, and epinephrine is converted to metanephrine. These metabolites can then be oxidatively deaminated by MAO to 3-methoxy-4-hydroxy mandelic acid (VMA). *(Katzung, p. 82)*

139. **(B)** Neostigmine in this example potentiates the muscarinic effects of acetylcholine. *(Katzung, p. 101)*

140. **(A)** The exogenous administration of acetylcholine is competitively inhibited by atropine so that muscarinic responses do not occur with the large acetylcholine dose. The presence of neostigmine allows acetylcholine to penetrate to the adrenal gland, resulting in epinephrine release and the stimulation of ganglia, resulting in the release of norepinephrine (active at adrenergic sites) and acetylcholine (blocked by atropine). *(Katzung, p. 102)*

141. **(C)** Phentolamine will eliminate the alpha$_1$-induced vasoconstriction, leaving the combined beta$_1$ and beta$_2$ activity (classic epinephrine reversal). *(Katzung, p. 140)*

142. **(E)** After the administration of phentolamine, only the beta-adrenergic response remains. Administration of a nonselective blocking agent will eliminate both the beta$_1$- and beta$_2$-adrenergic responses, that is, cardiac stimulation and skeletal muscle vasodilation, respectively. *(Katzung, p. 146)*

143. **(A)** The stimulation of alpha$_1$, alpha$_2$, beta$_1$, and beta$_2$ will give this classic epinephrine response. *(Katzung, p. 128)*

144. **(D)** The stimulation of alpha$_1$, alpha$_2$, and beta$_1$ will give this classic norepinephrine response. Vasodilation in skeletal muscle beds is not present with norepinephrine. *(Katzung, p. 128)*

145. **(B)** Isoproterenol, the classic nonselective beta-adrenergic agonist will stimulate both beta$_1$ (heart) and beta$_2$ (skeletal muscle vascular beds) to give this classic response. *(Katzung, p. 128)*

146. **(E)** The stimulation of alpha$_1$-adrenergic receptors by this agent, which is not inactivated by the usual processes, will result in a prolonged increase in blood pressure. *(Katzung, p. 128)*

147. **(D)** Bretylium has local anesthetic activity. It concentrates in adrenergic nerve endings and inactivates the transport of norepinephrine out of the nerve. *(Katzung, p. 80)*

148. **(E)** Simulation of the receptor on the effector will initiate a cascade of biochemical events, resulting in an action determined by the tissue cells (e.g., contraction of vascular smooth-muscle cells). *(Katzung, p. 80)*

149. **(G)** Indirect-acting adrenergic amines, the prototype being tyramine, enter the nerve ending and release norepinephrine from a "cytoplasmic storage" area. This "pool" is readily depleted and tachyphylaxis occurs. *(Katzung, p. 80)*

150. **(F)** Auto receptors of the alpha$_2$ type activate a negative feedback mechanism that inhibits norepinephrine release from the adrenergic nerve endings. *(Katzung, p. 80)*

151. **(K)** The activation of nicotinic N_M receptors located on skeletal muscle neuromuscular endplates results in opening of sodium and potassium channels and depolarization. *(Katzung, p. 83)*

152. **(I)** Formation of inositol 1,4,5-triphosphate (IP$_3$) and diacylglycerol (DAG) result in increased intracellular calcium. A similar process occurs in postsynaptic effector cells through alpha$_1$ receptor activation. *(Katzung, p. 83)*

153. **(F)** In the renal vascular bed, the administration of low-dose dopamine will selectively vasodilate and result in increased renal perfusion as a consequence of adenylyl cyclase activation. *(Katzung, p. 83)*

154. **(D)** The activation of adenylyl cyclase in bronchial and vascular smooth muscle as a consequence of stimulating beta$_2$ receptors results in relaxation. *(Katzung, p. 83)*

155. **(L)** The primary ganglionic receptor eliciting an excitatory postsynaptic potential (EPSP) in ganglia of the sympathetic or parasympathetic divisions of the autonomic nervous system occurs as a consequence of activation N_N receptors and the opening of sodium and potassium channels on the postganglionic neuron. *(Katzung, p. 83)*

156. **(E)** Stimulation of postsynaptic beta receptors on lipocytes results in an activation of adenylyl cyclase and increased cAMP. *(Katzung, p. 83)*

CHAPTER 3

Drugs Acting on the Central Nervous System
Questions

DIRECTIONS (Questions 157 through 251): Each of the numbered items or incomplete statements in this section is followed by answers or by completions of the statement. Select the ONE lettered answer or completion that is BEST in each case.

157. A 36-year-old man with a history of seizures is scheduled to undergo surgery for a hernia. You are asked to select a general anesthetic agent for this surgical event. The most appropriate choice is

(A) enflurane
(B) nitrous oxide
(C) propofol
(D) sevoflurane
(E) thiopental

158. The pharmacodynamic mechanism of action of general anesthetic agents is most likely related to

(A) depression of spontaneous and evoked neuronal activity
(B) hypopolarization of neurotransmitter-gated ion channels
(C) increased duration of opening of nicotinic receptor–activated cation channels
(D) inhibition of gamma-aminobutyric acid A ($GABA_A$) receptor chloride ion channels
(E) their oil/water partition coefficient

159. Which of the following general anesthetic agents has the shortest induction time?

(A) diethyl ether
(B) halothane
(C) isoflurane
(D) methoxyflurane
(E) nitrous oxide

160. The stage of general anesthesia characterized by breath holding, retching, and irregular respiration is

(A) stage I
(B) stage II
(C) stage III
(D) stage IV
(E) stage V

161. Concerns about toxicity with general anesthetic agents may most likely be related to

(A) a high incidence of malignant hyperthermia
(B) increased blood flow to the liver
(C) metabolism of general anesthetic agents
(D) storage in fat depots
(E) their carcinogenicity

162. The administration of an intravenous (IV) barbiturate is expected

(A) to have a slow (5 to 10 min) and smooth induction
(B) to cause tissue necrosis following extravasation
(C) to provide excellent analgesia
(D) to stimulate respiration
(E) to prevent laryngospasm

163. The anesthetic agent halothane

(A) decreases catecholamine-induced ar-rhythmias

(B) depresses the heart rate during anesthe-sia

(C) has an irritant effect on the tracheo-bronchial tree

(D) reduces stroke volume of the heart and decreases systemic blood pressure

(E) stimulates the sympathetic nervous sys-tem

164. The most appropriate agent for a patient with minimal circulatory reserve is

(A) diazepam

(B) halothane

(C) morphine

(D) nitrous oxide

(E) propofol

165. The side effect of propofol that is of concern is

(A) a feeling of impending doom following its use

(B) its cumulative effects causing delayed arousal

(C) its propensity to cause postoperative vomiting

(D) its slow recovery

(E) the production of acidosis in children

166. The action of which of the following IV anes-thetics can be reversed by flumazenil?

(A) etomidate

(B) fentanyl

(C) ketamine

(D) midazolam

(E) thiopental

167. General anesthetic–induced liver toxicity

(A) does not occur with halogenated agents

(B) is increased in compounds that are not metabolized

(C) occurs in the range of one in 1,000

(D) tends to occur in obese patients having multiple exposures to halothane

(E) usually resolves rapidly if specific anti-dotes are administered with the onset of toxicity

168. In the clinical use of general anesthetic agents

(A) chloroform is a stable agent for cardio-vascular surgery

(B) diethyl ether is still highly regarded and widely used

(C) methoxyflurane is reserved for long anesthetic procedures

(D) nitrous oxide is widely used because of its low toxicity and high potency

(E) the concept of "balanced anesthesia" is usually employed.

169. The term *general anesthesia* refers to

(A) amnesia and loss of consciousness pro-duced by ketamine

(B) analgesia produced by inhalational agents

(C) loss of consciousness and reflexes, anal-gesia, and skeletal muscle relaxation by inhaled agents

(D) the profound analgesia and loss of coop-eration when IV opioids are adminis-tered

(E) the use of a general group of drugs to produce loss of consciousness while minimizing potential harmful effects

170. Local anesthetic action

(A) is usually very acidic and requires bicar-bonate to activate it

(B) is dependent on metabolism to an active compound

(C) requires binding at the extracellular sur-face

(D) requires that agents have both lipophilicity and hydrophilicity

(E) results from agents that maintain nerves in the depolarized state

171. Nerves that are most sensitive to local anesthetic blockade are

(A) type A alpha proprioceptive fibers
(B) type A beta touch or pressure fibers
(C) type A delta pain or temperature
(D) type B preganglionic autonomic fibers
(E) type A gamma muscle spindles

172. Which of the following statements is true regarding blockade of fibers by local anesthetics?

(A) Fibers carrying touch are blocked before fibers carrying pain sensation.
(B) In fibers of the same diameter, unmyelinated fibers are blocked before myelinated fibers.
(C) Large myelinated fibers are blocked before small unmyelinated fibers.
(D) Motor fibers are blocked before pain fibers.
(E) Small fibers are blocked before large-diameter fibers.

173. Local anesthetic toxicity

(A) can be terminated by hypercapnia
(B) is decreased by administering compounds intravenously
(C) is due to progressive stimulation of cortical areas of the central nervous system (CNS)
(D) may be preceded by nystagmus when agents are administered intravenously
(E) occurs with progressive sedation and coma

174. Which of the following statements is true regarding allergic responses to local anesthetic agents?

(A) Allergic responses occur after administration of amides.
(B) Allergic responses occur after administration of esters.
(C) It is the metabolite of the amide structure that confers allergic response.

(D) The metabolite of the ester is responsible for allergic responses.

175. Which of the following statements is true regarding blockade of sodium channels?

(A) Lidocaine acts to block the channels from the outside of the membrane.
(B) Procaine blocks sodium channels by keeping the channels open.
(C) Saxitoxin blocks channels in a manner similar to procaine.
(D) Scorpion venoms act on the sodium channel to block sodium entry.
(E) Tetrodotoxin blocks sodium channels by binding near the extracellular surface.

176. Which of the following drugs is most effective in treating absence seizures?

(A) carbamazepine
(B) ethosuximide
(C) gabapentin
(D) phenobarbital
(E) phenytoin

177. Which of the following drugs exerts its anti-seizure activity mainly as a result of interference with ion conductance through sodium channels, which results in inhibition of high-frequency repetitive firing of neurons?

(A) carbamazepine
(B) clonazepam
(C) ethosuximide
(D) gabapentin
(E) phenobarbital

178. Valproate is effective in treating which of the following types of seizures?

(A) absence
(B) complex partial
(C) generalized tonic–clonic
(D) simple partial
(E) all of the above

179. Which of the following anticonvulsant drugs has been most associated with an idiosyncratic hepatotoxicity that is severe and has resulted in deaths, particularly in children?

    (A) carbamazepine
    (B) ethosuximide
    (C) phenytoin
    (D) primidone
    (E) valproate

180. Which of the following drugs probably exerts its antiseizure activity as a result of interference with conductance through calcium channels?

    (A) carbamazepine
    (B) ethosuximide
    (C) lamotrigine
    (D) phenytoin
    (E) primidone

181. What is the most likely mechanism of the antiseizure activity of phenytoin?

    (A) enhancement of the accumulation of GABA by inhibiting its biotransformation
    (B) enhancement of the accumulation of GABA by inhibition of GABA uptake into tissues
    (C) enhancement of the inhibitory effects of GABA by interaction with the GABA$_A$ receptor
    (D) interference with ion conductance through low-threshold calcium channels
    (E) interference with ion conductance through sodium channels

182. Which of the following drugs is (are) eliminated from the body mainly by excretion of the unchanged drug(s) in the urine?

    (A) carbamazepine
    (B) gabapentin
    (C) phenobarbital
    (D) phenytoin
    (E) all of the above

183. Which of the following drugs is most associated with gingival hyperplasia?

    (A) carbamazepine
    (B) ethosuximide
    (C) phenobarbital
    (D) phenytoin
    (E) valproate

184. Of the adverse reactions listed below, which is the most common dose-related effect observed during antiseizure therapy with carbamazepine?

    (A) diplopia
    (B) drowsiness
    (C) hepatic dysfunction
    (D) renal toxicity
    (E) skin rashes

185. Which of the following drugs is most readily metabolized to phenobarbital in the body?

    (A) carbamazepine
    (B) clonazepam
    (C) phenytoin
    (D) primidone
    (E) valproate

186. Valproate is known to inhibit the biotransformation of which of the following drugs?

    (A) carbamazepine
    (B) phenobarbital
    (C) phenytoin
    (D) all of the above
    (E) none of the above

187. Which of the following agents is most effective in stopping attacks of generalized tonic–clonic status epilepticus?

    (A) carbamazepine
    (B) diazepam
    (C) gabapentin
    (D) phenobarbital
    (E) phenytoin

188. Which of the following drugs is contraindicated in patients with a history of acute intermittent porphyria, variegate porphyria, hereditary coproporphyria, or symptomatic porphyria?

(A) carbamazepine

(B) ethosuximide

(C) phenobarbital

(D) phenytoin

(E) valproate

189. In the progressive depression of the CNS, the correct sequence is

(A) anesthesia–hypnosis–sedation–coma–death

(B) coma–hypnosis–sedation–coma–death

(C) hypnosis–sedation–anesthesia–coma–death

(D) hypnosis–sedation–anesthesia–sedation–coma–death

(E) sedation–hypnosis–anesthesia–coma–death

190. The distinction between an ideal sedative and an ideal hypnotic drug is

(A) sedative agents cause greater depression of the CNS than hypnotic agents

(B) sedative agents produce a reduction in cognitive functions while hypnotic agents do not

(C) sedative agents produce a reduction of anxiety while hypnotic drugs produce restful sleep

(D) sedative agents produce a state from which the person is easily aroused while hypnotic agents produce a trancelike state

(E) there is little difference between the two; it is just a matter of dose, especially with the benzodiazepines

191. Which of the following agents differs significantly in its pharmacologic actions?

(A) diazepam

(B) glutethimide

(C) meprobamate

(D) pentobarbital

192. A 60-year-old man in good health comes to you complaining of daytime sleepiness. On taking a history you find that he is being treated for insomnia with a benzodiazepine, chlordiazepoxide. The most likely explanation for this problem is

(A) circulation time is reduced and the effects are due to a reduction in blood flow

(B) he has liver disease and his microsomal oxidase system is not functioning well

(C) his phase II reactions are suppressed due to kidney failure

(D) the chlordiazepoxide is being metabolized to an active compound

(E) this is a normal and expected process for a 60-year-old man—he is just aging

193. Sedative hypnotic agents are noted for causing enzyme induction. Which of the following agents is least likely to cause enzyme induction?

(A) ethanol

(B) lorazepam

(C) meprobamate

(D) pentobarbital

(E) phenobarbital

194. A patient comes to your office complaining of daytime sleepiness. On questioning you find that he has been taking a benzodiazepine in order to go to sleep at night. He is in the process of discontinuing the use of this agent but needs some assistance for the next week. The most appropriate agent to prescribe is

(A) alprazolam

(B) flurazepam

(C) lorazepam

(D) quazepam

(E) triazolam

195. A 24-year-old woman arrives in the emergency department (ED) accompanied by her roommate. The roommate states that the patient has been using drugs for sleeping and thinks that an overdose was taken. You administer flumazenil and she recovers. Three hours later you return to find her in a hypnotic state. The most reasonable explanation for this is

(A) an overdose of flumazenil was given and she is experiencing the effects of the overdose
(B) another antagonist should be administered
(C) flumazenil does not reverse the effects observed
(D) she is experiencing the effects of other drugs (polypharmacy)
(E) the half-life of flumazenil is short

196. The clinical advantages of using benzodiazepines is based on

(A) active metabolites are not formed
(B) the fact that they are effective with ethanol
(C) they are rapidly eliminated from the body
(D) they have a high therapeutic index
(E) very little amnesia is experienced

197. Benzodiazepines are noted for having a long duration of action. This is often due to the biotransformation to active metabolites. Which of the following agents is NOT metabolized to an active compound?

(A) chlorazepate
(B) chlordiazepoxide
(C) diazepam
(D) lorazepam
(E) prazepam

198. A 17-year-old female high school student is brought by friends to the ED in a state of acute ethanol intoxication. They state that she has been vomiting profusely. One of the most important approaches to management is to administer

(A) glucose
(B) phosphate
(C) potassium
(D) sodium
(E) thiamine

199. Naltrexone has been administered to alcoholics with the result that their desire for the use of alcohol decreased. In these studies, which of the following was observed?

(A) Individuals given disulfiram suffered liver damage if naltrexone was added.
(B) Individuals who relapsed were unable to control their drinking.
(C) Naltrexone alone caused opioid receptor responses when patients drank alcohol.
(D) Patients resisted drinking, but once they started they drank more.
(E) The subjective high was increased when alcohol was ingested in the presence of naltrexone.

200. The management of methanol intoxication involves all of the following EXCEPT

(A) administration of folic acid
(B) administration of IV ethanol
(C) alkalinization with bicarbonate
(D) hemodialysis
(E) use of activated charcoal

201. The toxicity of methanol is mainly due to

(A) carbon dioxide
(B) conversion to ethanol
(C) formaldehyde
(D) formic acid
(E) methanol itself

202. Treatment of alcohol withdrawal should NOT include

(A) maintaining potassium and magnesium balance
(B) phenothiazines

(C) short-acting benzodiazepines in patients with liver disease

(D) the use of long-acting benzodiazepines

(E) thiamine administration

203. Your patient is concerned that his wife may be pregnant and they routinely have large parties at their home, where considerable amounts of alcohol are consumed by all present. He wonders if the child he suspects is on the way will suffer from a condition he has heard about called fetal alcohol syndrome. He wants to know what signs he should look for in the child once it is born. You tell him that fetal alcohol syndrome is characterized by

(A) a flattened face

(B) accelerated body growth

(C) an enlarged head

(D) major joint anomalies

(E) usually occurs only if drinking occurred late in pregnancy

204. The use of blood alcohol concentrations has both clinical and legal implications. Blood alcohol levels that cause emesis are

(A) 50 to 100 mg/dL

(B) 100 to 200 mg/dL

(C) 200 to 300 mg/dL

(D) 300 to 400 mg/dL

(E) >500 mg/dL

205. The ingestion of alcohol resulting in blood concentrations of 100 mg/dL may result in

(A) depletion of the liver of lipids

(B) greater intoxication in men than women

(C) premature labor

(D) ultrastructural heart damage

(E) vasoconstriction

206. The primary pathway for metabolism of ethanol involves

(A) alcohol dehydrogenase

(B) alcohol oxidase

(C) aldehyde dehydrogenase

(D) carbonic anhydrase

(E) microsomal ethanol oxidizing system (MEOS)

207. The effectiveness of levodopa

(A) is blocked by inhibiting dopa-decarboxylase

(B) can be prolonged by administering a catechol-O-methyltransferase (COMT) inhibitor

(C) is improved by administering centrally acting dopa decarboxylase inhibitors

(D) is increased by administering levodopa in combination with dopa

(E) inhibits the action of monoamine oxidase (MAO)

208. The use of antimuscarinic drugs in Parkinson's disease

(A) is most effective in eliminating the bradykinesia associated with the disease

(B) is most effective if large doses are administered initially

(C) leads to excessive salivation

(D) may be contraindicated in patients taking tricyclic antidepressants (TCAs)

(E) often causes urinary urgency

209. Dopaminergic therapy in the management of parkinsonian patients

(A) appears to be most effective in patients who do not respond well to levodopa

(B) is best managed initially with a nonergot dopamine agonist

(C) is easily managed with ergot derivatives as first-line agents

(D) is ineffective once on–off phenomena begin to occur

(E) results in the conversion of the agonist to compounds that block transport into the CNS

210. Gastrointestinal side effects of levodopa

(A) are mainly due to local irritation of the stomach and small intestine

(B) are reduced by administering phenothiazines as antiemetics

(C) can be minimized by taking the drug in one morning dose rather than divided doses

(D) occur in about 80% of patients when taken without a peripheral decarboxylase inhibitor

(E) should not be managed with antacids since these compounds reduce the effectiveness of levodopa

211. Side effects of levodopa therapy include

(A) accentuation of on–off phenomena if dietary intake of protein is reduced

(B) arrhythmias serious enough to discontinue the drug in most patients with heart disease

(C) behavorial effects, which are more common in patients on levodopa alone

(D) chorea, which can be successfully treated with pharmacologic agents

(E) dyskinesis, which tends to be more common in patients on concomitant decarboxylase inhibitor therapy

212. The pharmacotherapy of Parkinson's disease

(A) is best managed by administering low doses and gradually increasing the dose

(B) relieves all clinical features of the disease except the bradykinesia

(C) should include attention to dosing with meals to decrease irritation

(D) with a dopamine agonist tends to increase the fluctuations seen with levodopa

(E) with levodopa results in 80 to 90% of patients responding very well

213. Which of the following statements is true regarding a drug-induced parkinsonian-like tremor?

(A) MPTP (1-methyl-4-phenyl-1,2,5,6-tetrahydropyridine) may be effective in relieving this type of drug-induced tremor.

(B) Phenothiazines are noted for causing this type of tremor.

(C) Stimulation of dopamine receptors due to reserpine-induced depletion is the mechanism of this effect.

(D) The tremor induced by most drug therapy is not reversible.

(E) This type of side effect responds well to levodopa therapy.

214. Which of the following agents owes most of its antipsychotic activity to an active metabolite of the parent drug?

(A) clozapine

(B) haloperidol

(C) loxapine

(D) molindone

(E) thioridazine

215. Which of the following side effects of antipsychotic agents is characterized by feelings of restlessness and a compelling need to be in constant motion?

(A) acute dystonia

(B) akathisia

(C) neuroleptic malignant syndrome (NMS)

(D) parkinsonism

(E) tardive dyskinesia

216. Extrapyramidal side effects of antipsychotic agents are most likely due to the blockade of which of the following types of receptors?

(A) adrenergic $alpha_1$

(B) cholinergic M_1

(C) dopaminergic D_2

(D) $GABA_A$

(E) serotonergic $5-HT_2$

217. Blockade of which of the following types of receptors is most closely related to the antipsychotic effects of antipsychotic agents?

(A) adrenergic alpha$_1$
(B) adrenergic alpha$_2$
(C) dopaminergic D$_1$
(D) dopaminergic D$_2$
(E) muscarinic M$_1$

218. Which of the following conditions is most likely to be a troubling adverse reaction to phenothiazines?

(A) cardiac arrhythmias
(B) hepatic dysfunction
(C) megaloblastic anemia
(D) orthostatic hypotension
(E) thrombocytopenia

219. Which of the following neurological reactions to antipsychotic agents is rare but potentially fatal, and its manifestations may include a coarse tremor, catatonia, hyperthermia, stupor, and unstable pulse and blood pressure?

(A) acute dystonia
(B) akathisia
(C) neuroleptic malignant syndrome (NMS)
(D) parkinsonism
(E) tardive dyskinesia

220. Which of the following neurological side effects of antipsychotic agents may manifest soon after administration of the drug as facial grimacing, torsion of the neck or back due to muscle spasm, spasm of tongue muscles, or abnormal eye movements?

(A) acute dystonia
(B) akathisia
(C) NMS
(D) parkinsonism
(E) tardive dyskinesia

221. Which of the following antipsychotic agents has the greatest potential of producing bone marrow suppression or agranulocytosis in patients?

(A) clozapine
(B) haloperidol
(C) molindone
(D) olanzapine
(E) risperidone

222. Which of the following processes or enzyme activities is not inhibited by lithium ions?

(A) calcium-activated, phospholipid-dependent protein kinase C (PKC) activity
(B) inositol monophosphatase activity
(C) release of dopamine from nerve terminals
(D) release of norepinephrine from nerve terminals
(E) release of serotonin from nerve terminals

223. Which of the following agents has the smallest therapeutic index in terms of its potential for producing serious concentration-dependent toxic reactions?

(A) haloperidol
(B) lithium
(C) loxapine
(D) olanzapine
(E) quetiapine

224. Which of the following agents has the best evidence supporting its effectiveness for long-term prevention of recurrences of mania and bipolar depression?

(A) carbamazepine
(B) lithium
(C) lorazepam
(D) risperidone
(E) valproate

225. Which of the following antipsychotic agents has the least potential for producing extrapyramidal side effects in patients?

(A) clozapine

(B) haloperidol

(C) molindone

(D) pimozide

(E) risperidone

226. In treating depressed individuals, the generally accepted principle is to

(A) employ other agents to reduce the side effects

(B) intervene with a large dose and continue until relief is observed

(C) recognize that there is a standard dose that should not be exceeded

(D) start with a large dose and allow tolerance to develop

(E) start with a small dose and continue until relief or the maximum tolerated dose is reached

227. In considering the antidepressant drug classes, which class has the greatest potential to cause death if taken in excessive quantities?

(A) MAO inhibitors (MAOIs)

(B) second-generation drugs

(C) selective serotonin reuptake inhibitors (SSRIs)

(D) third-generation drugs

(E) TCAs

228. Which of the following pairs of antidepressant drugs is most dangerous?

(A) MAOIs–fermented foods

(B) second-generation antidepressants–beer or wine

(C) SSRIs–indirectly acting sympathomimetic amines

(D) TCAs–alcohol

(E) tricyclics–SSRIs

229. The predominant theory that explains how antidepressants relieve depression is

(A) a general enhanced activity of serotonin

(B) depletion of adrenergic amines in the CNS

(C) reduction of the effectiveness of serotonin

(D) the amine hypothesis

(E) there is no clear relationship between serotonin and depressant or antidepressant action

230. The serotonin syndrome

(A) is characterized by hyperthermia, muscle rigidity, and changes in vital signs

(B) is due to a combination of third-generation antidepressants and non-sedating antihistamines

(C) is usually caused by a lack of serotonin in the synapse leading to myoclonus

(D) results from the combination of SSRIs and acetylcholine

(E) will pass within an hour as long as the individual so afflicted maintains a prone position

231. MAOIs used to treat depression

(A) are more effective if a selective MAO-B inhibitor is used

(B) are toxic only if dopamine accumulates in the nerve endings

(C) cause irreversible blockade of MAO

(D) produce and increase in the first-pass metabolism to toxic intermediates

(E) result in the accumulation of norepinephrine but not serotonin in the synapse

232. Therapy with antidepressants

(A) might be discontinued slowly after 6 to 9 months of therapy if this was the first episode

(B) will not be required long term in most patients suffering from depression

(C) should be continued long term if a patient responds quickly and satisfactorily to drug therapy

(D) should not exceed 1 year

(E) usually results in a major lessening of depression within 3 to 4 days

233. Which of the following peptides has the greatest affinity for mu opioid receptors?

(A) endomorphin I

(B) leu-enkephalin

(C) met-enkephalin

(D) preprodynorphin

(E) prepro-opiomelanocortin (POMC)

234. Tolerance develops to many of the effects of opioids. Two effects that do not develop or develop very little tolerance are

(A) analgesia and miosis

(B) cough suppression and respiratory depression

(C) miosis and constipation

(D) respiratory depression and analgesia

(E) sedation and euphoria

235. Patients who are ambulatory may experience

(A) an increase in the perception of pain but a decreased sensory component

(B) direct depression of cardiac contractile force development

(C) mydriasis

(D) relaxation of the biliary tract

(E) stimulation of the chemoreceptor trigger zone, resulting in vomiting

236. The phenomenon in which withdrawal of a drug results in physiologic changes is referred to as

(A) cross-tolerance

(B) direct toxicity

(C) physical dependence

(D) psychological dependence

(E) tolerance

237. Which of the following is the most rational use of morphine?

(A) IV administration for the relief of dyspnea in congestive heart failure

(B) maintaining a regular pattern of dosing at 4- to 6-hour intervals

(C) relief of sharp intermittent pain

(D) suppression of cardiovascular reflexes in surgery

(E) suppression of angiotensin-converting enzyme (ACE)-induced cough

238. The metabolism of which of the following opioid analgesics to a toxic metabolite has led to a reduction in its use?

(A) codeine

(B) dilaudid

(C) fentanyl

(D) meperidine

(E) methadone

239. For the relief of pain, morphine is most effective in

(A) patients with head injuries

(B) pregnant patients

(C) relieving constant pain

(D) treating patients with neuropathic pain

(E) relieving intermittent sharp pain

240. The pharmacodynamic process in which response to a drug requires increasingly larger doses to achieve the desired effect is referred to as

(A) abuse

(B) addiction

(C) misuse

(D) psychological dependence

(E) tolerance

241. In the early stages of alcohol consumption, college students learn to stand up slowly and not to change positions rapidly. This process is

(A) behavioral tolerance

(B) functional tolerance

(C) metabolic tolerance

(D) physiologic dependence

(E) psychological dependence

242. Treatment of patients dependent on opioids (e.g., heroin, morphine) provides a challenge since the recidivism rate is very high. Methadone maintenance is effective in some patients because

(A) detoxification from methadone is easier than from other opioids

(B) it blocks the action of street drugs

(C) it provides a constant high, thus eliminating drug-seeking behavior

(D) they become dependent on methadone providing a "hold" on them

(E) they must be "clear" (drug free) before starting therapy with methadone

243. Withdrawal reactions from barbiturates and sedative hypnotics are related to the half-life of the drug. Compounds in these categories are often grouped as ultra-short, short, inter-mediate, or long acting. Which of the following categories presents the most difficult or most intense withdrawal process?

(A) $t_{1/2} = <4$ hours

(B) $t_{1/2} = 8$ to 24 hours

(C) $t_{1/2} = 48$ to 96 hours

(D) $t_{1/2} = >96$ hours

244. Sedative–hypnotic drugs, which include ethanol, the barbiturates, and the benzodi-azepines, have similar abuse patterns. A unique phenomenon that develops in some benzodiazepine abusers is

(A) paresthesias and headaches

(B) physiologic dependence

(C) rapid withdrawal

(D) the "Mickey Finn"

(E) therapeutic dose dependence

245. CNS stimulants are common drugs of abuse. Worldwide, the most common CNS stimulant is

(A) amphetamine

(B) caffeine

(C) cocaine

(D) methamphetamine

(E) nicotine

246. In the current climate of drug abuse, young people attend parties known as raves. At these parties the drug of choice is referred to as ecstasy. This drug is a(n)

(A) amphetamine

(B) barbiturate

(C) benzodiazepine

(D) hallucinogen

(E) nicotine derivative

247. LSD (lysergic acid diethylamide), mescaline, and psilocybin are all agents that have psychotomimetic effects. These agents

(A) are not associated with dependence or physiologic withdrawal

(B) have approximately the same potency

(C) have markedly different psychotomimetic effects

(D) lose their effectiveness if administered orally

(E) produce a great deal of tolerance

248. Treatment of hallucinogenic drug overdose with

(A) antimuscarinic agents can be managed with a direct-acting cholinergic agonist

(B) any drug in this class should be managed by tapering off the drug

(C) LSD should be managed with phenothiazines

(D) phencyclidine (PCP) can be partially managed by nasogastric suction

(E) PCP is best managed by alkalinization of the urine

249. All of the following are true about inhalant drugs of abuse EXCEPT

   (A) amyl nitrite is associated with widespread and life-threatening methemoglobinemia

   (B) chloroform has been associated with demyelination of white matter in chronic users

   (C) fluorocarbons may cause sudden death due to ventricular arrhythmias

   (D) the principle users of these agents are teenage boys of lower socioeconomic groups

   (E) these agents are widely available as industrial solvents

250. Steroid dependence

   (A) does not result in a withdrawal syndrome when drugs are discontinued

   (B) is rather easily detected by routine laboratory screening

   (C) may express itself as increased aggression

   (D) results from the euphoria these drugs produce

   (E) while considered negative may result in elevation of high-density lipoprotein (HDL) and reduction in low-density lipoprotein (LDL) cholesterol

251. Marijuana

   (A) can be classified with the amphetamines since its effects mimic this drug class

   (B) consists of three active cannabinoids: cannabidiol, tetrahydrocannabinol (THC), and cannabinol

   (C) has had effective use as a bronchodilator in the management of chronic obstructive pulmonary disease (COPD) and bronchial asthma

   (D) is a substitute for alcohol in those who regularly use this agent

   (E) is most effectively used for treating nausea and vomiting if taken prophylactically

DIRECTIONS (Questions 252 through 283): Each group of questions in this section consists of groups of lettered headings followed by lists of numbered words or phrases. For each numbered word or phrase, select the ONE lettered heading that is most closely associated with it. Each lettered heading may be selected once, more than once, or not at all.

Questions 252 through 257

Match each drug with the appropriate description.

   (A) benzocaine
   (B) bupivacaine
   (C) cocaine
   (D) lidocaine
   (E) procaine
   (F) tetracaine

252. An ester-type compound with relatively short duration of action

253. An ester local anesthetic agent with high potency and long duration of action

254. An agent reserved for topical use only

255. No vasoconstrictor is needed with this agent due to its natural structure.

256. No vasoconstrictor is used with this agent when it is employed as an antiarrhythmic.

257. A long-acting and potent amide-type local anesthetic

Questions 258 through 262

Match the appropriate item with its description.

   (A) beta-carbolines
   (B) BZ_1 (benzodiazepine receptor subtype 1)
   (C) BZ_2
   (D) duration of channel opening
   (E) endozepines
   (F) flumazenil
   (G) frequency of channel opening
   (H) pentobarbital

258. A sedative–hypnotic agent of the benzodi-azepine type would be expected to act on the chloride channel to increase _____.

259. Naturally occurring molecule that has affinity for benzodiazepine receptors

260. An inverse agonist

261. A benzodiazepine antagonist

262. Zaleplon and zolpidem have selectivity for this site.

Questions 263 through 269

    (A) amantadine
    (B) benztropine
    (C) bromocriptine
    (D) glutamate
    (E) pramipexole
    (F) selegiline
    (G) tocopherol
    (H) tolcapone

263. Large multicenter trials have found no evidence of benefit in treating Parkinson's disease with this agent.

264. A dopamine agonist that is considered a non-ergot derivative

265. In addition to its effectiveness in parkinsonism, it also has therapeutic efficacy in hyperprolactinemia.

266. Inhibits the metabolism of dopamine

267. An antiviral drug with effectiveness in parkinsonism

268. Effective in relieving the tremor and rigidity of parkinsonism

269. A neurotransmitter associated with parkinsonism

Questions 270 through 272

Match each agent with the appropriate description.

    (A) bupropion
    (B) fluoxetine
    (C) imipramine
    (D) phenelzine
    (E) venlafaxine

270. MAOI

271. SSRI

272. TCA

Questions 273 through 276

Match each drug with the appropriate clinical description.

    (A) amitriptyline
    (B) bupropion
    (C) desipramine
    (D) fluoxetine
    (E) fluvoxamine
    (F) mirtazapine
    (G) trazodone

273. Significant side effects include sedative and antimuscarinic action.

274. Inhibits serotonin uptake selectively with a notable absence of antimuscarinic or sedative side effects

275. Has considerable sedative action but little or no antimuscarinic side effects

276. A unique third-generation agent that does not block the amine pump for norepinephrine or serotonin

Questions 277 through 283

    (A) apomorphine

    (B) codeine

    (C) dextromethorphan

    (D) dilaudid

    (E) fentanyl

    (F) heroin

    (G) loperamide

    (H) methadone

    (I) morphine

    (J) naltrexone

277. Useful for treating diarrhea with minimal or no danger of producing opioid dependence

278. Used to induce vomiting

279. Used for the withdrawal of patient with opioid dependence

280. A very potent analgesic administered intravenously or by patch

281. An excellent cough suppressant devoid of opioid-induced dependence

282. May be expected to induce withdrawal when administered to an individual with opioid dependence

283. Should be administered to a patient who appears in the ED with pinpoint pupils and respiratory depression

Answers and Explanations

157. **(D)** Sevoflurane is the best choice since propofol and thiopental are used for induction or short procedures. Nitrous oxide is not a complete agent. Enflurane may cause seizures and is not used in a patient with a history of epilepsy. *(Katzung, pp. 427, 430)*

158. **(A)** While there is correlation between anesthetic potency and lipid solubility (Meyer–Overton Principle), more recent evidence indicates that depression of neuronal activity is more probably the mechanism of action. This process results from stimulation of $GABA_A$ receptor chloride ion channels, hyperpolarization of neurotransmitter-gated ion channels, and/or decreased duration of opening of nicotinic receptor–activated cation channels. *(Katzung, p. 425)*

159. **(E)** The speed of induction is inversely related to the blood:gas partition coefficient. Nitrous oxide has the lowest partition coefficient and is the agent with the fastest onset. *(Katzung, pp. 422–423)*

160. **(B)** The excitement stage (II) occurs with the loss of consciousness, and general anesthetic practice is to minimize this stage. Surgical anesthesia is stage III, medullary depression is stage IV, and stage I is the stage of analgesia and amnesia. *(Katzung, pp. 420–422)*

161. **(C)** When a high degree of metabolism occurs, fluoride ions are released with a greater incidence of toxicity. These agents are not proven carcinogens. They decrease blood flow to the liver, and they do not produce a high degree of malignant hyperthermia. This

latter condition is a relatively rare genetic disorder. *(Katzung, pp. 428–429)*

162. **(B)** The solution of sodium pentothal has a pH of over 10, and extravasation leads to tissue damage. It can cause laryngospasm, has a rapid (10-sec) induction period, depresses respiration, and may even be antianalgesic, causing exaggerated pain responses. *(Katzung, pp. 430–431)*

163. **(B)** Halothane depresses the heart but does not change systemic vascular resistance. It does not evoke a compensatory increase in sympathetic nervous system activity but does sensitize the heart to catecholamines. It does not usually cause respiratory depression. *(Katzung, pp. 426–427)*

164. **(C)** In individuals requiring cardiac surgery or in patients in whom circulatory reserve is minimal, opioid analgesics provide good circulatory support. *(Katzung, p. 431)*

165. **(E)** This agent has a very fast onset of action, can be used repeatedly, and still provides a rapid recovery. It has antiemetic properties. *(Katzung, p. 432)*

166. **(D)** Midazolam is a benzodiazepine with a slow onset and recovery but has the advantage of having a specific antidote for reversal of its action. *(Katzung, p. 430)*

167. **(D)** Halogenated agents like halothane have an incidence of liver toxicity of about 1:20,000, and there is no specific antidote or treatment for halothane hepatitis. Multiple

exposures in obese individuals increases susceptibility. Metabolism releases toxic halogens. *(Katzung, p. 428)*

168. **(E)** Inhaled anesthetic agents are rarely used alone because greater safety can be obtained with combinations of agents. Diethyl ether has vanished due to its explosive nature, as has methoxyflurane due to its nephrotoxicity. Nitrous oxide has very low potency, and chloroform produces fatal arrhythmias. *(Katzung, pp. 429–430)*

169. **(C)** The term *general anesthesia* refers to the production of a state in which analgesia, amnesia, loss of consciousness, inhibition of sensory and autonomic reflexes, and loss of skeletal muscle tone exists. No agent currently in use accomplishes all of these characteristics to a satisfactory level. Supplementation and combinations of agents are needed for the greatest safety and the least chance of causing harm. *(Katzung, p. 419)*

170. **(D)** Local anesthetics require a balance between hydro- and lipophilicity in order to be soluble for injection and to penetrate to the inside of the nerve cell membrane where they block the sodium channel. *(Katzung, p. 438)*

171. **(D)** Type B and type C fibers are the most sensitive to local anesthetic blockade. *(Katzung, p. 440)*

172. **(E)** Small fibers, which carry pain, are preferentially blocked, but in fibers of the same diameter myelinated fibers are blocked first. *(Katzung, p. 440)*

173. **(D)** Hyperventilation or administration of oxygen is helpful in reversing the inhibition of convulsant activity of intravenously administered local anesthetic agents. A prominent sign of impending seizures may be nystagmus or circumoral numbness. *(Katzung, pp. 441–442)*

174. **(D)** *p*-Aminobenzoic acid, the metabolite of the ester structure, is responsible for the aller-

gic response. The amides are not metabolized in the same manner. *(Katzung, p. 443)*

175. **(E)** All of the compounds listed act on the sodium channel. The local anesthetics lidocaine and procaine bind to the intracellular side of the channel, while tetrodotoxin and saxitoxin bind extracellularly. Scorpion toxin binds in the channel and keeps it open. *(Katzung, p. 439)*

176. **(B)** Ethosuximide is effective against absence seizures, probably as a result of its effect to reduce low-threshold calcium currents in thalamic neurons. The other drugs listed in this item—phenytoin, carbamazepine, gabapentin, and phenobarbital—are effective in treating partial seizures and, with the possible exception of gabapentin, are effective against generalized tonic–clonic seizures. *(Katzung, pp. 408–409)*

177. **(A)** Carbamazepine interferes with sodium conductance by prolonging the inactive state of sodium channels in a manner similar to phenytoin. *(Katzung, pp. 397–398, 400–401)*

178. **(E)** Valproate has possibly the broadest spectrum of antiseizure activity of any of the currently available drugs and can be used for the treatment of all of the seizure types listed in this item. *(Katzung, p. 410)*

179. **(E)** The risk of idiosyncratic hepatotoxicity due to valproate is greatest in children under 2 years of age and in those taking multiple medications. *(Katzung, p. 411)*

180. **(B)** The ion channels inhibited by ethosuximide are the low-threshold calcium channels in thalamic neurons. *(Katzung, p. 408; Hardman et al., p. 475)*

181. **(E)** Phenytoin prolongs the inactive state of sodium channels and thereby interferes with sustained high-frequency repetitive firing of action potentials. *(Katzung, pp. 397–398)*

182. **(B)** Gabapentin is not metabolized in the body and does not induce hepatic drug me-

tabolizing enzymes, but rather is eliminated from the body by renal mechanisms. The other drugs listed in this item are metabolized in the liver. *(Katzung, p. 406)*

183. **(D)** Phenytoin causes gingival hyperplasia to some degree in most patients receiving the drug. *(Katzung, p. 400)*

184. **(A)** Diplopia and ataxia are the most common dose-related adverse reactions observed during therapy with carbamazepine. Drowsiness may occur at higher doses than usually used in antiseizure therapy. Hepatic dysfunction is unusual. *(Katzung, p. 402)*

185. **(D)** Phenobarbital is cleared more slowly than primidone, and therefore it slowly accumulates to higher levels than the parent compound, reaching therapeutic concentrations during prolonged therapy. *(Katzung, p. 404)*

186. **(D)** Valproate is known to inhibit the biotransformation of several drugs, including those listed in this item, resulting in higher steady-state concentrations of these drugs in the body. *(Katzung, pp. 410–411)*

187. **(B)** Diazepam is given intravenously to stop the attacks of generalized tonic–clonic status epilepticus, a life-threatening emergency. Some physicians prefer lorazepam, which may be somewhat longer acting. Since the antiseizure effect of the benzodiazepines does not last long, a longer-acting antiseizure agent, such as phenytoin, is usually also given to suppress seizure activity in the longer term. *(Katzung, pp. 415–416)*

188. **(C)** Barbiturates are absolutely contraindicated in patients with a history of any of the conditions listed in this item because these drugs enhance porphyrin synthesis. *(Katzung, p. 378)*

189. **(E)** Continual depression of the CNS occurs in a dose-dependent manner with the older sedative–hypnotic agents like barbiturates. The benzodiazepines are safer in that they do not have a linear relationship with dose and depression. *(Katzung, pp. 364–365)*

190. **(C)** The goal of these widely prescribed and used agents is to produce a decrease in anxiety with no or little effect on motor or cognitive function (sedatives) or to produce a "natural" sleep-like state (hypnotics). *(Katzung, p. 364)*

191. **(A)** Glutethimide, meprobamate, and pentobarbital are virtually indistinguishable. They all have barbiturate pharmacologic properties. The benzodiazepines (diazepam) are less apt to cause CNS depression at high doses. *(Katzung, pp. 364–365)*

192. **(D)** While kidney or liver disease is a possibility, it is well recognized that benzodiazepines are metabolized to active compounds that have half-lives longer than their parent compounds. This is most likely the cause of his current difficulty. *(Katzung, p. 367)*

193. **(B)** The benzodiazepines do not alter hepatic drug-metabolizing enzymes with continued use. *(Katzung, p. 369)*

194. **(E)** Flurazepam and quazepam are metabolized to active compounds while lorazepam has a long duration of action. Of the two remaining compounds, the shortest duration of action is with triazolam. *(Katzung, pp. 368, 376)*

195. **(E)** The half-life of flumazenil is of the order of 1 hour (0.7 to 1.3 hours). It is necessary to monitor the patient for repeated administration of this antagonist. *(Katzung, pp. 373–374)*

196. **(D)** The high therapeutic index is the biggest advantage of these agents. They should not be used with ethanol, they are slowly eliminated, they are metabolized to active compounds, and amnesia is a major component of their action. *(Katzung, p. 375)*

197. **(D)** Lorazepam is an agent that has active metabolites. It is conjugated and renally excreted. See chart in reference. *(Katzung, p. 368)*

198. **(B)** While all of the above are possible choices, phosphate loss (exaggerated by glu-

cose administration) may lead to poor wound healing, neurologic deficits, and increased risk of infection. *(Katzung, pp. 389–390)*

199. **(A)** Both naltrexone and disulfiram are hepatotoxins and should not be used concomitantly. All of the other statements provided the opposite result. *(Katzung, pp. 391–392)*

200. **(E)** The use of activated charcoal is ineffective in methanol intoxication. *(Katzung, pp. 392–393)*

201. **(D)** It is the formate derivatives that produce the toxicity. *(Katzung, p. 392)*

202. **(B)** Phenothiazines have the potential of inducing seizures. One of the major objectives of managing alcohol withdrawal is to prevent seizures, arrhythmias, and delirium. *(Katzung, p. 390)*

203. **(A)** The characteristics of fetal alcohol syndrome (associated with alcohol ingestion during the first trimester of pregnancy) include a flattened face, retarded body growth, microcephaly, minor joint abnormalities, and mental retardation. *(Katzung, p. 388)*

204. **(C)** The lowest levels (50 mg/dL) are associated with sedation or a high, followed by impaired motor function (100 mg/dL), then emesis (200 mg/dL), then coma (300 mg/dL), and finally respiratory depression and death (> 500 mg/dL). *(Katzung, p. 384)*

205. **(D)** Ethanol at these levels definitely causes myocardial damage at the ultrastructural level. It also causes vasodilation, relaxation of smooth muscle (premature labor inhibition), the deposition of fats in the liver, and greater intoxication in women than men. *(Katzung, pp. 384–385)*

206. **(C)** The primary pathway is the conversion of alcohol to an aldehyde. *(Katzung, p. 383)*

207. **(B)** Selective inhibitors of COMT prolong the action of levodopa by inhibiting its peripheral metabolism. The COMT metabolite of levodopa competes with the carrier for levodopa in the CNS, and inhibiting this enzyme improves central penetration of levodopa. "On time" is increased. *(Katzung, p. 470)*

208. **(D)** Agents like TCAs, which have considerable cholinergic side effects, may be expected to exacerbate the complications of anticholinergic side effects, including dry mouth and urinary retention. Low-dose therapy and increasing levels slowly, is most effective in improving the tremor and rigidity but has little effect on the bradykinesia. *(Katzung, p. 471)*

209. **(B)** Dopamine agonists will prolong the effectiveness of therapy when used as first-line agents and may be effective in preventing on–off sequences. They are not ergot derivatives like the older agents. *(Katzung, p. 468)*

210. **(D)** The use of decarboxylase inhibitors reduces the gastrointestinal side effects from approximately 80% to 20%. This, along with taking the drug in divided doses or using antacids 30 to 60 minutes before taking levodopa, reduces the nausea and vomiting due to chemoreceptor trigger zone (CTZ) stimulation. *(Katzung, p. 465)*

211. **(E)** Reduction of dietary protein reduces side effects. The arrhythmias usually do not warrant discontinuation of therapy, and the behavorial effects are more common in patients taking carbidopa. Chorea is not successfully managed with drugs. *(Katzung, pp. 466–467)*

212. **(A)** About one third of patients respond very well if low doses are administered, with a slow progression of the dose as needed for control. Bradykinesia is a feature, which is relieved, and the adverse effects of levodopa can be minimized by taking before meals (30 to 60 min) or by combining it with a dopamine agonist to decrease fluctuations in response. *(Katzung, p. 465)*

213. **(B)** The tremor induced by drugs like phenothiazines or reserpine is reversible following cessation of drug therapy. It is not re-

versed by levodopa, which may worsen the condition. MPTP causes severe parkinsonism. *(Katzung, pp. 472–473)*

214. **(E)** Thioridazine is converted in the body to mesoridazine, a major metabolite that is more potent than the parent compound. *(Katzung, p. 480)*

215. **(B)** Akathisia typically occurs within 5 to 60 days after onset of therapy and is one of the more disturbing side effects of the antipsychotic agents. It has not yet been reproduced in animal models that might facilitate its study. *(Hardman et al., pp. 501–502; Katzung, p. 488)*

216. **(C)** Extrapyramidal side effects are probably caused by blockade of dopaminergic receptors in the basal ganglia. Antipsychotic agents with low potential for producing extrapyramidal effects have relatively low affinity for D_2 receptors. *(Hardman et al., pp. 492–493; Katzung, pp. 482, 488)*

217. **(D)** There is a strong correlation between the antipsychotic potency of drugs and their ability to block D_2 receptors in the limbic system of the brain. Some of the atypical antipsychotic agents also block cortical 5-HT_2 receptors with high affinity. *(Katzung, pp. 482–483; Hardman et al., pp. 493–496)*

218. **(D)** Orthostatic hypotension, probably caused by blockade of adrenergic alpha$_1$ receptors, may cause syncope and falls in affected patients. *(Hardman et al., p. 500; Katzung, p. 484)*

219. **(C)** In NMS, serum creatine kinase may be elevated and myoglobinemia may be present. Care usually consists of discontinuation of the offending drug and supportive care. Use of dantrolene or bromocriptine may also be helpful. *(Hardman et al., p. 502; Katzung, p. 489)*

220. **(A)** Acute dystonia usually responds well to anticholinergic antiparkinsonian drugs administered parenterally. *(Hardman et al., pp. 500–501; Katzung, p. 488)*

221. **(A)** Bone marrow suppression and agranulocytosis have been reported for other antipsychotic agents, but they are particularly prevelant with clozapine, for which the incidence approaches 1% within several months of therapy. *(Hardman et al., pp. 503–504; Katzung, pp. 486, 488)*

222. **(E)** Depolarization-provoked release of serotonin from nerve terminals is not inhibited by the lithium ion and may even be increased in the limbic system. Lithium ion is known to interfere with several biological processes and enzyme activities, but its exact mechanism as a mood-stabilizing agent remains unknown. *(Hardman et al., pp. 507–508; Katzung, pp. 490–491)*

223. **(B)** The therapeutic index for lithium may be as low as 2 or 3. Because of this low therapeutic index, determination of serum or plasma levels is essential during therapy. Concentrations much above the therapeutic range can cause acute intoxication characterized by gastrointestinal symptoms, tremor, ataxia, sedation, coma, and convulsions. *(Hardman et al., pp. 509–510; Katzung, pp. 492–493)*

224. **(B)** Whereas all of the agents listed in this item may be useful in managing patients with mania or bipolar illness, lithium is the agent with the best evidence supporting its effectiveness as long-term therapy aimed at preventing recurrences of mania and bipolar depression. *(Hardman et al., pp. 511–512; Katzung, pp. 491–492)*

225. **(A)** Clozapine has a relatively low potential for producing extrapyramidal effects, but its potential for producing blood dyscrasias is higher than other commonly used antipsychotic agents. *(Hardman et al., pp. 488–489, 503; Katzung, p. 486)*

226. **(E)** Since the effective dose of antidepressants can vary widely, the common practice is to start with a low dose and increase it gradually until side effects become overwhelming or the depression lifts. *(Katzung, pp. 507–508)*

227. **(E)** TCAs are very dangerous, especially in patients with suicidal tendencies. Com-

pounds should be prescribed in limited quantities or entrusted to a family member. *(Katzung, p. 509)*

228. **(A)** It is well recognized that fermented foods and beer or wine should be avoided by patients on MAOIs. *(Katzung, p. 508)*

229. **(E)** There are numerous theories to explain how antidepressants work; however, it appears that no clear relationship exists between serotonin and the effectiveness of antidepressants. *(Katzung, pp. 498, 504)*

230. **(A)** The combination of an SSRI and an MAOI may result in a dangerous increase in serotonin in the synapse, producing a serotonin syndrome characterized by hyperthermia, muscle rigidity, and changes in vital signs. *(Katzung, p. 505)*

231. **(C)** MAO-A inhibition with the older agents is irreversible and results in an accumulation of norepinephrine, serotonin, and dopamine in the synapses of neurons. Tyramine-containing foods are not metabolized by the usual first-pass process and hence enter the bloodstream, resulting in excessive release of adrenergic amines. *(Katzung, p. 505)*

232. **(A)** The treatment of this condition depends on the history of the disease. If it is the first episode, discontinuation slowly after a 6- to 9-month treatment period is reasonable. Repetitive episodes usually require indefinite treatment. *(Katzung, pp. 507–508)*

233. **(A)** The endogenous opioid peptides (previously called endorphins) with the highest affinity is endomorphin I (also endomorphin II). The enkephalins have higher affinity for delta opioid receptors. Preprodynorphin and POMC are precursor proteins. *(Katzung, pp. 513–514)*

234. **(C)** Many of the effects of opioids develop tolerance but not constipation, miosis, convulsions, and antagonist actions. *(Katzung, p. 520)*

235. **(E)** Opioids directly activate the CTZ. However, they produce miosis, contraction of the biliary tract, and reduction of both sensory and affective pain response while having minimal or no effect on cardiac contractile force development. *(Katzung, p. 520)*

236. **(C)** Physical dependence accompanies the repeated use of opioids. *(Katzung, p. 524)*

237. **(A)** While the mechanism is not understood, the use of morphine in pulmonary edema is remarkable. Morphine dosing with patient-controlled analgesia is more effective than a strict dosing pattern. This drug relieves constant pain better than sharp pain, and it does not suppress cardiovascular reflexes. Nonaddicting agents should be used to suppress cough. *(Katzung, pp. 522–523)*

238. **(D)** Meperidine is metabolized to normeperidine. Its accumulation results in seizures. *(Katzung, p. 526)*

239. **(C)** Rather than sharp pain, it is constant pain, such as associated with cancer, that is most effectively relieved by morphine. Morphine is contraindicated in closed head injuries because it increases intracranial pressure. In pregnant patients it may depress the fetus or cause dependence in the fetus. Neuropathic pain is best treated with other agents. *(Katzung, pp. 522–523)*

240. **(E)** The term *tolerance* simply means that more drug is needed to achieve the same desired effect. This can be clinical effectiveness and is not necessarily linked to inappropriate use of the drug. Compensatory responses may mitigate the drug's pharmacodynamic action. *(Katzung, p. 532)*

241. **(A)** Behavioral tolerance is the learned ability to compensate for the effect of a drug. In this case, if alcohol inhibits locomotor activity, exerting that activity in a slow manner can mask the effect of alcohol to depress motor function. *(Katzung, p. 532)*

242. **(D)** The advantage of methadone is its long duration of action and its oral effectiveness in preventing the high from intravenous street-acquired opioids. Since the individual is de-

pendent on the agent, the avoidance of withdrawal will bring him or her back to the treatment center for continued availability of the drug. *(Katzung, p. 535)*

243. **(B)** The most rapidly evolving and most difficult to treat withdrawal syndrome occurs with agents that have a half-life of 8 to 28 hours (secobarbital). The short-acting compounds (thiobarbiturates) cannot be taken repeatedly, the long-acting compounds (phenobarbital) have built-in tapering, and the agents with 48- to 96-hour half-lives (flurazepam) produce a long but less severe withdrawal. *(Katzung, pp. 535–536)*

244. **(E)** Some patients who continually use benzodiazepines do not increase the dose but will enter withdrawal if the drug is discontinued. This use is not associated with physiologic dependence, but it does produce paresthesias, weight loss, headaches, and changes in perception. *(Katzung, p. 536)*

245. **(B)** Many people do not consider caffeine to be a drug since it comes from a natural product, but a withdrawal syndrome is recognized in heavy coffee drinkers (6 cups per day). *(Katzung, p. 537)*

246. **(A)** Methylenedioxymethamphetamine (MDMA, ecstasy) is the drug that is in wide abuse among high school and college students. They take it with large amounts of water, and the environment is kept at a very low temperature. Methamphetamine is known as "speed." *(Katzung, p. 537)*

247. **(A)** These three agents, which are indistinguishable in effect, have the same effect orally or intravenously and do not produce tolerance or withdrawal. The effective doses vary 5,000-fold—LSD, 1 µg/kg; psilocybin, 250 µg/kg; mescaline, 5 to 6 mg/kg. *(Katzung, p. 541)*

248. **(D)** Since PCP is secreted back into the stomach, nasogastric suction may be helpful. Acidification of the urine increases elimination of PCP. Phenothiazines may worsen the toxic effects of LSD. Antimuscarinic agents

can be treated with indirect-acting cholinergic agonists. *(Katzung, pp. 541–542)*

249. **(A)** While amyl nitrite may cause an occasional instance of methemoglobinemia, very few significant adverse effects of this agent have been reported, even though it is widely abused. *(Katzung, p. 545)*

250. **(C)** Behavioral changes (aggression, libido, mood, psychotic behavior) may result from steroid abuse, which is expensive and difficult to detect with routine laboratory tests. Those who take these compounds usually do so for bodybuilding (increase in muscle mass and strength), not for euphoria. Continued use results in unfavorable lipid profiles (increased LDL and decreased HDL). *(Katzung, p. 546)*

251. **(B)** The three active components of marijuana begin with cannabidiol, which is metabolized to THC and on to cannabinol. The age of plants can be estimated based on the relative amounts of these cannabinoids. The drug is often taken with alcohol, it is effective as an antiemetic during nausea, and it may cause bronchoconstriction. *(Katzung, pp. 542–544)*

252. **(E)** Procaine is rapidly hydrolyzed by plasma cholinesterase. *(Katzung, p. 437)*

253. **(F)** Tetracaine is about 16 times the potency of procaine, and it has a long duration of action. *(Katzung, p. 437)*

254. **(A)** Benzocaine is reserved for surface use only. *(Katzung, p. 437)*

255. **(C)** Cocaine blocks uptake of norepinephrine into nerve endings, prolonging its duration of action by reducing blood flow to the area. *(Katzung, pp. 89, 443)*

256. **(D)** Lidocaine is used as a class II antiarrhythmic agent and is marketed in packages with blue marking to distinguish it from preparations containing vasoconstrictors (red package). *(Katzung, pp. 235, 443)*

257. (B) Similar to tetracaine, an ester-type local anesthetic, bupivacaine, an amide, is a long-acting agent with about 16 times the potency of procaine. *(Katzung, p. 437)*

258. (G) Barbiturates increase the duration of opening while benzodiazepines increase the frequency of opening of the chloride channels. *(Katzung, p. 370)*

259. (E) Endozapines are nonbenzodiazepine molecules that facilitate GABA-mediated chloride channel gating. *(Katzung, p. 370)*

260. (A) Agents of this type, referred to as inverse agonists, produce anxiety and seizures. *(Katzung, p. 371)*

261. (F) Flumazenil selectively blocks benzodiazepine receptors analogous to naloxone and the opioid receptors. It does not reverse barbiturates, meprobamate, or ethanol. *(Katzung, p. 370)*

262. (B) The receptors for benzodiazepines are heterogenous and additional molecular characterization is needed. However, selectivity for BZ_1 has been demonstrated for zaleplon and zolpidem. *(Katzung, p. 374)*

263. (G) The scavenger of free radicals (vitamin E, tocopherol) was suggested as a beneficial treatment to slow progression of Parkinson's disease, but trials have not supported this hypothesis. *(Katzung, p. 471)*

264. (E) Mild parkinsonism is benefited by this agonist, which has preferential affinity at D_3 receptors and allows the dose of levodopa to be reduced. Pramipexole does not have the serious adverse effects associated with ergot compounds. *(Katzung, p. 469)*

265. (C) This D_2 agonist is effective in treating endocrinologic disorders in doses lower than used for parkinsonism. *(Katzung, p. 468)*

266. (F) Selegiline is a selective inhibitor of monoamine oxidase B. It is effective in retarding the breakdown of dopamine in the brain. *(Katzung, p. 469)*

267. (A) Amantadine has limited effectiveness in parkinsonism. It may be helpful in eliminating all of the unfavorable effects of parkinsonism, but benefits often do not last more than two weeks. *(Katzung, p. 470)*

268. (B) Antimuscarinic agents have a considerable number of side effects and have little effect on the bradykinesia. *(Katzung, p. 471)*

269. (D) Glutamate excess may be linked to parkinsonism, and studies under way are testing the effectiveness of glutamate antagonists. *(Katzung, p. 472)*

270. (D) Tranylcypromine and phenelzine are MAOIs. The effectiveness of these agents persists even after the drug is eliminated from the body. *(Katzung, p. 503)*

271. (B) Fluoxetine is an SSRI. It has little effect on norepinephrine but effectively inhibits the removal of serotonin from the nerve ending. *(Katzung, p. 505)*

272. (C) Imipramine is named a tricyclic antidepressant because of its characteristic three-ring nucleus and the fact that it is effective in treating depression. It blocks the uptake of both norepinephrine and serotonin. *(Katzung, p. 499)*

273. (A) This TCA has considerable side effects. *(Katzung, p. 504)*

274. (E) Both bupropion and fluvoxamine have an absence of antimuscarinic action and sedative action. It is fluvoxamine that is a blocker of the serotonin amine pump. *(Katzung, p. 504)*

275. (G) The SSRI trazodone has little or no antimuscarinic activity. *(Katzung, p. 504)*

276. (F) Mirtazapine has antihistaminic and $alpha_2$ blocking activity and causes weight gain. It has almost no sexual side effects but does cause considerable sedation. *(Katzung, p. 505)*

277. (G) Both loperamide and diphenoxylate are compounds with a low likelihood for abuse because of poor solubility in the case of diphenoxylate (also combined with atropine) or inability to penetrate the brain in the case of loperamide. *(Katzung, p. 527)*

278. **(A)** Apomorphine produces emesis by stimulating receptors in the floor of the fourth ventricle of the brain called the CTZ (chemotrigger-receptor-zone). It is a highly vascular area where many drugs that cause nausea and vomiting act. It must be injected. Caution should be used with this compound since it causes respirator depression. *(Hardman et al., p. 249)*

279. **(H)** The conversion of opioid-dependent individuals to methadone and then withdrawing them from this agent is based on the principle that the longer duration of action of methadone produces a longer but more tolerable withdrawal sequence. The drug is also effective orally. *(Katzung, p. 526)*

280. **(E)** This group of strong opioid agonists includes sufentanil, alfentanil, remifentanil, and fentanyl. They have a greater potency and pharmacokinetics that make them effective for short-term use. *(Katzung, p. 526)*

281. **(C)** The dextro isomer of levorphanol is essentially free of analgesic activity, respiratory depression, and addictive properties, and it produces minimal constipation. It is available in over-the-counter preparations for cough suppression. *(Katzung, p. 528)*

282. **(J)** Naloxone, naltrexone, and nalmefene are agents with groups substituted on the nitrogen in the 17 position. This makes them have high affinity for the mu opioid–binding sites, where they compete effectively with other opioids. However, they are pure antagonists, so they do not activate the receptor. Caution needs to be exerted when using these agents because they have short half-lives and quickly wear off. *(Katzung, p. 528)*

283. **(J)** The combination of pinpoint pupils and respiratory depression is characteristic of opioid overdose. Often, these signs are accompanied by needle marks. Pure antagonists are very effective in reversing the opioids. *Caution:* The duration of action of the antagonists is shorter than that of the agonists. *(Katzung, pp. 525, 528)*

CHAPTER 4

Drugs Affecting the Cardiovascular System
Questions

DIRECTIONS (Questions 284 through 348): Each of the numbered items or incomplete statements in this section is followed by answers or by completions of the statement. Select the ONE lettered answer or completion that is BEST in each case.

284. Antihypertensive agents lower blood pressure by altering anatomic control sites. Which of the following statements is correct?

    (A) Antihypertensive drug therapy requires patients to maintain consistent drug therapy over many years.
    (B) Antihypertensive therapy usually results in noted improvement in most patients suffering from elevated blood pressure.
    (C) Cardiac output is most effectively managed by lowering venomotor tone.
    (D) Inhibiting the renin–angiotensin system has not proven effective in long-term lowering of peripheral resistance.
    (E) The use of combination drugs to manage hypertension makes it difficult to maintain efficacy with decreased toxicity.

285. The benefit of compounds like pindolol over propranolol is based on the fact that

    (A) pindolol is a partial agonist
    (B) pindolol is long acting
    (C) pindolol is selective
    (D) pindolol is short acting
    (E) propranolol is a membrane depressant

286. In selecting a calcium channel blocker for the treatment of hypertension, which of the following is a correct statement?

    (A) Antihypertensive calcium channel blockers exert their effect on venous smooth muscle.
    (B) The dihydropyridines are more selective vasodilators than verapamil.
    (C) The short-acting compounds like nifedipine are most effective as antihypertensive agents.
    (D) These agents are used in abnormal cardiac rhythms in twice the antihypertensive dose.
    (E) Verapamil and diltiazem are less effective in depressing cardiac output.

287. Angiotensin-converting enzyme (ACE) inhibitors

    (A) are usually potentiated by nonsteroidal anti-inflammatory drugs (NSAIDs)
    (B) have a side effect that is described as an altered sense of taste
    (C) have excellent effectiveness in patients with hypovolemia due to diuretics
    (D) may be of particular benefit in patients who are pregnant
    (E) may cause hypokalemia when they are used with potassium-sparing diuretics

288. The advantage of losartan over captopril is that

(A) losartan is a more selective compound
(B) losartan is rapidly metabolized to an inactive compound
(C) losartan is safe to use in pregnancy
(D) losartan will inhibit non–ACE-generated angiotensin
(E) losartan blocks bradykinin metabolism

289. Digoxin-induced arrhythmias are most likely due to

(A) alterations in threshold potential
(B) blockade of potassium channels
(C) calcium overload
(D) slow heart rates
(E) stimulation of sodium ion flux

290. Abnormalities in cardiac conduction that give rise to abnormal cardiac rhythms are known as

(A) changes in maximum membrane potential
(B) disturbances in impulse formation
(C) early afterdepolarizations
(D) generation defects
(E) reentry phenomena

291. A 45-year-old woman presents with an arrhythmia, and the treating physician prescribes quinidine. She is rushed to the emergency department (ED) with an excessively high ventricular rate. This might have been prevented by

(A) administration of a beta-adrenergic blocker after the quinidine
(B) administration of a cholinesterase inhibitor after quinidine
(C) amiodarone
(D) atropine administration to suppress vagal activity
(E) pretreatment with a low dose of digoxin to increase vagal tone

292. In patients with renal failure, torsade de pointes may result due to accumulation of the metabolite of

(A) amiodarone
(B) metoprolol
(C) procainamide
(D) quinidine
(E) verapamil

293. The antiarrhythmic agent with broad-spectrum activity (i.e., it could be classed in all four categories) is

(A) amiodarone
(B) metoprolol
(C) procainamide
(D) quinidine
(E) verapamil

294. The major result of the Cardiac Arrhythmia Suppression Trial (CAST) was

(A) abnormal cardiac rhythms, especially premature ventricular contractions, increase the risk of sudden death
(B) all abnormal electrical activity in the myocardium should be suppressed
(C) even asymptomatic arrhythmias should be treated to prevent their progressive development
(D) mortality from cardiac arrhythmias was markedly reduced by administration of flecainide
(E) no drug therapy should be instituted unless there is a reasonable assumption of benefit

295. The administration of which of the following compounds may be expected to cause an initial tachycardia?

(A) amiodarone
(B) bretylium
(C) procainamide
(D) quinidine
(E) verapamil

296. In patients with atrial arrhythmias resistant to DC cardioversion, the administration of which of the following agents results in a very high success rate of restoring normal rhythm?

    (A) amiodarone
    (B) bretylium
    (C) ibutilide
    (D) quinidine
    (E) sotalol

297. The cardiac glycoside digoxin

    (A) enters into the enterohepatic circulation
    (B) is eliminated by the kidney
    (C) is extensively metabolized by the liver
    (D) is metabolized to a more active compound
    (E) must be injected intravenously since it has low bioavailability

298. Low doses of cardiac glycosides administered to patients results in

    (A) a decreased PR interval
    (B) accumulation of calcium ion
    (C) delayed afterdepolarizations
    (D) slowed heart rate
    (E) tachycardia

299. Primary changes in the electrocardiogram (ECG) induced by digoxin include

    (A) accentuation of the T wave
    (B) increasing the PR interval
    (C) QT interval shortening
    (D) shortening of the PR interval
    (E) widening of the QRS complex

300. The cardiac inotropic actions of digoxin are

    (A) a consequence of Na^+/K^+ adenosine triphosphatase (ATPase) inhibition
    (B) a result of decreased calcium ion
    (C) due to accumulation of cyclic adenosine monophosphate (cAMP)

    (D) due to changes in the electrical properties of cardiac muscle cells
    (E) the result of beta-adrenergic stimulation

301. The major effects of cardiac glycosides on electrical activity of the heart include

    (A) a decrease in automaticity in the ventricular muscle
    (B) a decrease in effective refractory period in the atrial muscle
    (C) decreased conduction velocity in atrial muscle
    (D) increased conduction velocity in the atrioventricular (AV) node
    (E) shortened refractory period in the AV node

302. Extracardiac effects of digoxin include

    (A) a direct vasodilation and reduction of peripheral resistance
    (B) disorientation and hallucinations in the elderly
    (C) enhancement of visual acuity
    (D) inhibition of nausea and vomiting due to inhibition of the chemoreceptor trigger zone (CTZ) in the central nervous system (CNS)
    (E) reduction in breast size due to competition with estrogen for estrogen receptors

303. Changes in ions have marked influences on the action of digoxin. These actions include

    (A) decreased potassium leads to a reduction in digoxin toxicity
    (B) hypomagnesemia will be beneficial in treating digitalis intoxication
    (C) increased potassium leads to increased digoxin binding to tissues
    (D) magnesium will counter the cardiotoxicity of digoxin
    (E) the level of calcium ion is neutral when it comes to digitalis intoxication

304. Studies have shown that agents that decrease survival in treating chronic congestive heart failure (CHF)

   (A) are agents that increase intracellular cAMP
   (B) are associated with an increase in calcium in the myocardial cell
   (C) block the loss of potassium ion in the kidney
   (D) facilitate AV conduction
   (E) increase ventricular automaticity

305. Treatment of acute CHF is appropriately managed with

   (A) digoxin
   (B) inovasodilators
   (C) methylxanthines
   (D) oral administration of milrinone
   (E) selective beta$_1$ agonists

306. The combination of isosorbide dinitrate and hydralazine is appropriate

   (A) as first-line therapy for most patients with CHF
   (B) for heart failure complicated by ventricular arrhythmias
   (C) for the initial treatment of heart failure
   (D) for the long-term management of heart failure
   (E) in patients with ACE inhibitor intolerance

307. In chronic CHF, the use of beta-adrenergic agents is based on which of the following?

   (A) Beta-adrenergic blocking agents should not be used because they suppress contractile force development.
   (B) Beta blockers keep the heart from developing tachycardia.
   (C) Beta$_1$ selective antagonists prevent arrhythmias.
   (D) Beta$_1$ agonists are useful in maintaining cardiac output.
   (E) These agents inhibit the toxic effects of calcium channel–blocking agents.

308. Treatment of cardiac glycoside intoxication manifested by visual or gastrointestinal (GI) disturbances

   (A) includes reducing the dose, correcting electrolytes, and waiting one to two half-lives
   (B) includes the discontinuation of digoxin immediately and no further use of this agent
   (C) rarely requires the monitoring of serum digoxin levels
   (D) should include routine parenteral administration of potassium ion
   (E) with Fab antibody fragments may result in acute elevation of digoxin

309. In managing chronic CHF

   (A) aldosterone antagonists generally should be avoided
   (B) angiotensin II receptor blocker administration reduces mortality
   (C) calcium channel blockers are effective agents
   (D) patients who are on digoxin should be converted to ACE inhibitors
   (E) vasodilators are superior to ACE inhibitors

310. The half-life of digoxin

   (A) is 7 days
   (B) is reduced in patients suffering from renal failure
   (C) is short when compared with most pharmacologic agents
   (D) is such that it may require a week to stabilize a patient with maintenance doses
   (E) usually results in the need to reduce the initial dose to prevent toxicity

311. Cardiac glycosides

   (A) are considered steroid antagonists
   (B) are found in oleander, lily of the valley, and numerous plants
   (C) are inactive if the sugar portion of the molecule is removed

(D) are relatively nontoxic unless taken with fatty foods

(E) require a saturated lactone ring at position 17 for biologic activity

312. The HMG-CoA reductase inhibitors are not all active in the form administered clinically. Which of the following must be converted in the GI tract to an active compound?

(A) atorvastatin
(B) cerivastatin
(C) fluvastatin
(D) pravastatin
(E) simvastatin

313. In understanding the role of lipoproteins, one group of lipids is considered antiatherogenic. This group is

(A) chylomicrons
(B) high-density lipoproteins (HDLs)
(C) intermediate-density lipoproteins (IDLs)
(D) low-density lipoproteins (LDLs)
(E) very-low-density lipoproteins (VLDLs)

314. The National Cholesterol Education Program provides treatment guidelines for hypercholesterolemia. What is the desirable total cholesterol in an adult, assuming no other risk factors?

(A) < 130 mg/dL
(B) < 159 mg/dL
(C) < 200 mg/dL
(D) < 239 mg/dL
(E) < 240 mg/dL

315. In deciding to treat a patient with elevated cholesterol levels, secondary causes must first be eliminated. Which of the following will result in secondary hypercholesterolemia rather than secondary hypertriglyceridemia?

(A) alcohol ingestion
(B) diabetes mellitus
(C) early nephrosis
(D) estrogens
(E) isotretinoin

316. Patients with reduced HDL levels should be treated with

(A) atorvastatin
(B) clofibrate
(C) gemfibrozil
(D) niacin
(E) pravastatin

317. Triglyceride levels in patients may be lowered by dietary manipulation. A dietary method of lowering triglycerides is

(A) a diet severely restricted to 10 g/d of fat
(B) administration of a "statin"
(C) administration of homocysteine
(D) eating vegetable oils rich in omega-6 fatty acids
(E) omega-3 fatty acid ingestion

318. The pharmacokinetics of nitroglycerin make its route of administration important. It is administered

(A) by patch to provide long-term efficacy
(B) in high doses to prevent the development of tolerance
(C) intravenously
(D) orally to enhance metabolism to an active metabolite
(E) sublingually to avoid the "first-pass" effect in the liver

319. The orally effective form of nitro-vasodilator agents is

(A) amyl nitrite
(B) glyceryl trinitrate
(C) isosorbide dinitrate
(D) nitric oxide
(E) nitroglycerin

320. The effectiveness of nitroglycerin in angina pectoris is primarily due to

(A) a reflex decrease in sympathetic nervous system activation

(B) arterial vasodilation

(C) redistribution of coronary blood flow

(D) relaxation of the veins with an increase in capacitance (decreased preload)

(E) the negative inotropic effect on myocardial cells

321. Nitroglycerin relaxes

(A) all three forms of muscle

(B) cardiac muscle

(C) skeletal muscle

(D) smooth muscle

(E) smooth muscle and cardiac muscle

322. The use of organic nitrites has proved effective in

(A) erectile dysfunction

(B) GI spasticity

(C) relaxing bile ducts in managing gallstones

(D) treating bronchial asthma

(E) all of the above

323. Your patient has been experiencing chest pain on exertion. One of his friends told him that he has been taking a drug for hypertension and that it is very effective in lowering blood pressure. The friend suggests that your patient try some of the drug: "It won't hurt anything and it may save the expense of a doctor's visit." He tries the agent and experiences severe chest pain, worse than before. The explanation of this phenomenon may be

(A) "coronary steal" occurred

(B) a nitrate arteriolar dilator should have been used

(C) reflex vasoconstriction occurred

(D) the drug suppressed the heart

(E) venous dilation occurred

324. The term *Blue Monday disease* refers to

(A) a withdrawal phenomenon experienced by workers physically dependent on organic nitrates

(B) color alterations in patients with glaucoma

(C) organic nitrate inactivation of hemoglobin

(D) the throbbing headaches caused by loss of tolerance

(E) the use of organic nitrates in closed head injury

325. Erectile dysfunction has been treated by numerous agents over the centuries. The effectiveness of these agents depends on intact parasympathetic innervation and

(A) a bladder or urethral irritant (Spanish fly)

(B) a reduction in the levels of cyclic guanosine monophosphate (cGMP)

(C) an $alpha_2$ antagonist to relax nonvascular smooth muscle in the penis

(D) an inhibitor of phosphodiesterase isoform 5

(E) blockade of prostaglandin E_1 (PGE_1)

326. The clinical effectiveness of organic nitrates is based on which of the following pairs?

(A) angina of effort–increased coronary blood flow

(B) recurrent rest angina–increased coronary blood flow

(C) unstable angina–decreased platelet aggregation

(D) variant angina–decreased myocardial oxygen demand

(E) variant angina–decreased myocardial contractile force

327. Diltiazem

(A) effectively relaxes skeletal muscle

(B) has a greater ratio of cardiac effects relative to vascular smooth muscle effects

(C) inhibits the contraction of venous smooth muscle rather than arteriolar smooth muscle

(D) is considered to be in the dihydropyridine group of calcium channel blockers

(E) is more effective in relaxing vascular smooth muscle than inhibiting cardiac muscle

328. Which of the following statements about calcium channel blockers is true?

(A) Calcium channel blockers may increase morbidity following subarachnoid hemorrhage.

(B) Calcium channel blockers stimulate insulin release.

(C) Some reports indicate that calcium channel blockers limit infarct size.

(D) Stimulus secretion coupling is effectively inhibited in many tissues by calcium channel blockers.

(E) The short-acting calcium channel blockers exert a very low degree of negative inotropic effects.

329. A 49-year-old man is suffering from hypertension, and he has a history of atrial tachycardia. In selecting a calcium channel blocker to manage the tachycardia, the most appropriate agent would be

(A) amlodipine
(B) isradipine
(C) nifedipine
(D) propranolol
(E) verapamil

330. A 55-year-old woman presents with angina pectoris and she is placed on a beta-adrenergic blocking agent. The rationale for the use of a beta blocker is

(A) that an increase in end-diastolic volume will increase contractile force development

(B) production of a decrease in heart rate, blood pressure, and contractility

(C) production of an increase in myocardial oxygen demand

(D) production of coronary artery vasodilation

(E) redistribution of coronary blood flow to ischemic areas

331. A 46-year-old man who is overweight and in a high-pressure executive position has been treated with a beta-adrenergic blocking agent (propranolol) for episodes of angina pectoris. The diagnosis is angina of effort. Lately, the effectiveness of propranolol has been less than desired, and he is also complaining that he feels tired. The most appropriate approach to therapy would be to

(A) add metoprolol to the regimen

(B) add nifedipine to the regimen

(C) advise him to quit his job and find another profession

(D) increase the dose of propranolol

(E) revise the therapy to combine a beta blocker, a calcium channel blocker, and a nitrate

332. The effect of which of the following agents can be reversed by administration of vitamin K?

(A) clopidogrel
(B) eptifibatide
(C) tirofiban
(D) unfractionated heparin
(E) warfarin

333. Which of the following drugs decreases the anticoagulant effects of warfarin by inducing hepatic enzymes that transform the anticoagulant in the body?

(A) amiodarone
(B) cimetidine
(C) fluconazole
(D) metronidazole
(E) rifampin

334. Which of the following agents is an inhibitor of fibrinolysis?

(A) aminocaproic acid
(B) dalteparin
(C) danaparoid
(D) lepirudin
(E) phytonadione

335. Which of the following agents inactivates fibrin-bound thrombin in thrombi?

(A) dalteparin
(B) danaparoid
(C) dipyridamole
(D) lepirudin
(E) urokinase

Questions 336 through 341

Refer to Figure 4.1 below for questions 336 through 341.

336. In a 60-year-old patient with marked kidney disease, the choice of an agent to treat edema would be one that acts at site _____.

337. In a 24-year-old man suffering from a head injury received in a motorcycle accident, the most appropriate agent to employ for reduction of intracranial pressure would be a compound acting at site _____.

338. Hypercalcemia requiring the elimination of calcium ion is effectively managed by administering diuretics that act at site _____.

339. Compounds acting at site _____ were widely used to manage hypertension and are still effective agents in many (two thirds) patients. They may cause potassium depletion.

340. A patient with ascites and severe edema as a consequence of advanced liver disease would be expected to respond well to an agent acting at site _____.

341. Drugs acting at site _____ prevent the reabsorption of sodium bicarbonate.

342. Many patients routinely consume NSAIDs for the management of fever, headache, or muscle aches due to inflammation. NSAIDs will inhibit the action of all of the following EXCEPT

(A) aldosterone antagonists
(B) carbonic anhydrase inhibitors
(C) mannitol
(D) thiazides
(E) triamterene

343. Diuresis refers to the elimination of

(A) magnesium ion
(B) potassium ion

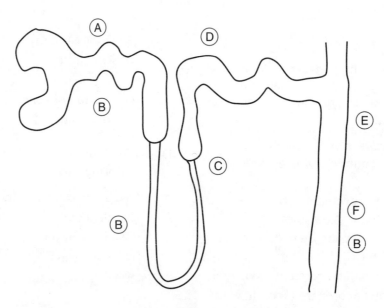

Figure 4.1

(C) sodium ion

(D) urine volume

(E) water

344. In a patient with altered hearing, the agent most likely to exacerbate this deficit is

(A) acetazolamide

(B) furosemide

(C) hydrochlorothiazide

(D) mannitol

(E) spironolactone

345. The appropriate description of the mechanism of action of antidiuretic hormone (ADH) in promoting urine flow is

(A) enzyme inhibition

(B) interference with hormone receptors

(C) interference with proteins responsible for potassium ion transport

(D) interference with proteins responsible for sodium transport

(E) prevention of water reabsorption

346. In a patient with CHF being treated with digoxin

(A) a high intake of sodium should be avoided

(B) diuretic therapy should be limited to loop diuretics

(C) diuretics will prevent arrhythmias

(D) oral mannitol is the agent of choice if diuretics are employed

(E) potassium ion supplements should be administered routinely

347. Most diuretics have the potential to cause hypokalemia; however, in the presence of beta blockers or ACE inhibitors, hyperkalemia would be expected with the administration of

(A) acetazolamide

(B) furosemide

(C) hydrochlorothiazide

(D) mannitol

(E) spironolactone

348. In a 65-year-old man with benign prostatic hypertrophy (BPH), which of the following agents should be avoided?

(A) ADH antagonists

(B) carbonic anhydrase inhibitors

(C) loop diuretics

(D) osmotic diuretics

(E) potassium-sparing diuretics

DIRECTIONS (Questions 349 through 383): Each group of questions in this section consists of groups of lettered headings followed by lists of numbered words or phrases. For each numbered word or phrase, select the ONE lettered heading that is most closely associated with it. Each lettered heading may be selected once, more than once, or not at all.

Questions 349 through 356

From the list of sites of action of antihypertensive agents, match the statements below with the type of agent selected.

(A) beta receptors of the heart

(B) beta receptors of the juxtaglomerular cells

(C) alpha receptors of vessels

(D) ACE

(E) angiotensin receptors of vessels

(F) kidney tubules

(G) sympathetic ganglia

(H) sympathetic nerve terminals

(I) vascular smooth muscle

(J) vasomotor center

349. Agents acting at this site may cause an increase in bradykinin levels.

350. African-Americans respond better to agents acting at this site.

351. This group of agonists, characterized by clonidine, lower blood pressure by stimulating receptors to lower blood pressure.

352. Blockade of this site coupled with the action of beta blockers on the heart is most likely responsible for the hypotensive action of propranolol.

353. Reserpine and guanethidine produce antihypertensive action at this site.

354. Nonselective drug action at this site leads to excessive tachycardia.

355. The most common side effect of agents acting at this site is potassium depletion.

356. Carvedilol is an effective antihypertensive agent that acts nonselectively at beta-adrenergic receptors, but also acts at additional sites selectively. These sites are _____.

Questions 357 through 361

Antiarrhythmic drugs are traditionally classified on the basis of their dominant mechanism of action. Match the following agents with the most prominent effect in preventing arrhythmias.

(A) amiodarone
(B) lidocaine
(C) metoprolol
(D) quinidine
(E) verapamil

357. Blocks sodium channels and increases the duration of the action potential

358. Shortens the duration of the action potential and has local anesthetic activity

359. Inhibits catecholamine-induced arrhythmias

360. Markedly prolongs the action potential duration

361. Its antiarrhythmic action is dependent on calcium channel blockade.

Questions 362 through 368

Match the drug with its mechanism of action, its use, or its toxicity.

(A) colestipol
(B) gemfibrozil
(C) niacin
(D) simvastatin

362. Primarily employed in patients with elevated triglyceride levels

363. Inhibits the absorption of cholesterol bile acids

364. May have adverse effects on plasma levels of cardiac glycosides, fat-soluble vitamins, or thyroxine

365. A structural analog of 3-hydroxy-3-methyl-glutaryl coenzyme A (HMG-CoA) intermediate

366. Patients taking this agent often complain of uncomfortable flushing and itching.

367. Some patients experience muscle pain, tenderness, and weakness when given this agent.

368. Combination of this agent with simvastatin is the most efficacious treatment of familial combined hyperlipidemia.

Questions 369 through 374

Match each drug to the appropriate description.

(A) angiotensin I
(B) atrial natriuretic peptide (ANP)
(C) bradykinin
(D) endothelin (ET-I)
(E) substance P
(F) vasoactive intestinal peptide (VIP)
(G) vasopressin

369. An intravenous injection of this vasoactive peptide initially causes vasodilation followed by long-lasting vasoconstriction.

370. Participates in the physiologic regulation of sodium excretion

371. The vasodilator action of this compound is due to its action on arteries; it contracts veins.

372. Produced by the enzymatic action of renin

373. The physiologic role is to increase water reabsorption.

374. Relaxes airway and vascular smooth muscle and thought to be a modulator

Questions 375 through 383

For each pharmacological agent, select the statement that is most closely associated with it.

(A) The activated partial thromboplastin time (aPTT) is used to monitor the effect of this agent in patients.

(B) This agent blocks the gamma-carboxylation of glutamate residues in factors II (prothrombin), VII, IX, and X.

(C) This agent combines with proactivator plasminogen to form a complex that catalyzes the conversion of inactive plasminogen to active plasmin.

(D) This agent inhibits mainly activated factor X, but only slightly inhibits other clotting factors.

(E) This agent irreversibly acetylates cyclooxygenase, resulting in inhibition of the synthesis of thromboxane A_2.

(F) This agent reduces platelet aggregation by binding to the platelet IIb/IIIa receptor complex.

(G) This agent reduces platelet aggregation by irreversibly blocking the adenosine diphosphate (ADP) receptor on platelets.

375. Abciximab

376. Aspirin

377. Clopidogrel

378. Eptifibatide

379. Low-molecular-weight heparin

380. Streptokinase

381. Tirofiban

382. Unfractionated heparin

383. Warfarin

Answers and Explanations

284. (A) Compliance with antihypertensive therapy is difficult since patients are often asymptomatic and not readily convinced that medications that have undesirable side effects are beneficial in the long run. *(Katzung, p. 157)*

285. (A) The major benefit of pindolol is the fact that it, along with acebutolol and penbutolol, has intrinsic sympathomimetic tone. This effect results in less cardiac depression and may be of benefit in patients with reduced cardiac function. It also causes less hypertensive rebound when discontinued abruptly. *(Katzung, p. 167)*

286. (B) Verapamil is mainly used for its antiarrhythmic or antianginal effect, while dihydropyridine compounds are used as arteriolar vasodilators with less cardiac depressant action. The long-acting agents are less apt to cause toxicity due to a sudden drop in blood pressure. *(Katzung, p. 172)*

287. (B) The altered sense of taste is viewed by some as an unacceptable alteration of one of the pleasures of life. These agents may be inhibited by NSAIDs and are contraindicated in hypovolemic states and in pregnancy. In the presence of potassium-sparing diuretics, they may cause hyperkalemia. *(Katzung, p. 174)*

288. (D) Enzymes other than ACE are able to convert angiotensin I to angiotensin II. The angiotensin receptor blockers (losartan) will block this non-ACE generated angiotensin II. Losartan is contraindicated in pregnancy, is metabolized to an active metabolite, and does

not provide a selectivity advantage. *(Katzung, p. 174)*

289. (C) Digoxin inhibits Na^+-K^+ ATPase and increases calcium ion in the myocardial cell. This accumulation eventually leads to delayed afterdepolarizations. *(Katzung, p. 225)*

290. (E) The term *reentry* indicates that the impulse has been conducted through a pathway and that it can reexcite tissue previously depolarized. It is also referred to as a conduction or circus movement arrhythmia. *(Katzung, p. 227)*

291. (E) The use of digoxin to prevent quinidine-induced paradoxical tachycardia is well established. Prior administration of a calcium channel blocker or a beta-adrenergic blocker may also be effective. *(Katzung, p. 230)*

292. (C) The N-acetylation of procainamide produces NAPA (N-acetylprocainamide), which has class III antiarrhythmic activity. The accumulation of this metabolite in patients with renal failure is implicated in the development of torsade de pointes. *(Katzung, p. 231)*

293. (A) Amiodarone is considered a class III agent because of the prolongation of action potential duration, most likely due to potassium channel blockade. However, it also blocks sodium channels, noncompetitively blocks beta-adrenergic receptors, and inhibits calcium channels. *(Katzung, p. 234)*

294. (E) It was the assumption and the general practice that premature ventricular contractions should be suppressed since they may lead to the development of sudden death. The data indicated that a twofold increase in death occurred when treatment with flecainide was initiated. This led to the conclusion that there must be a reasonable assumption that risk will be outweighed by benefit. *(Katzung, p. 237)*

295. **(B)** Bretylium will inhibit the development of ventricular fibrillation. However, upon initial administration, it releases catecholamines and stimulates the heart rate. This action may precipitate ventricular arrhythmias. *(Katzung, p. 238)*

296. **(C)** The intravenous administration of ibutilide or dofetilide in patients resistant to electrical conversion of atrial arrhythmias to normal rhythm is very effective in achieving conversion. *(Katzung, p. 239)*

297. **(B)** Digoxin is fairly well absorbed after oral administration. It is mainly eliminated by the kidney. Digitoxin is mainly metabolized by the liver. *(Katzung, p. 205)*

298. **(D)** Low concentrations of cardiac glycosides increase parasympathomimetic activity. Sensitization of the baroreceptors, central vagal stimulation, and facilitation of muscarinic transmission all occur. *(Katzung, p. 207)*

299. **(B)** Cardiac glycosides increase the PR interval (vagal effect), shorten the QRS complex, and invert the T wave. *(Katzung, p. 207)*

300. **(A)** Inhibition of Na^+/K^+ ATPase results in an increase in calcium ion and an increase in contractile force development. *(Katzung, p. 206)*

301. **(B)** A primary effect of cardiac glycosides is to decrease the refractory period in atrial muscle, leading to atrial flutter or fibrillation. All of the other changes described occur in the opposite direction. *(Katzung, p. 207).*

302. **(B)** Digoxin, especially at toxic levels, may cause disorientation in the elderly, which may be confused with degeneration of central

nervous function. Other side effects include gynecomastia, an increase in nausea and vomiting, and alterations in yellow-green vision. The decrease in peripheral resistance is a consequence of reversal of compensatory mechanisms, not a direct effect of digoxin to relax blood vessels. *(Katzung, p. 208)*

303. **(D)** Magnesium can be used to decrease digitalis intoxication. Lower levels of potassium and increased levels of calcium contribute to increased toxicity. Monitoring of serum electrolytes is of great importance in using cardiac glycosides, especially when glycoside intoxication is suspected. *(Katzung, p. 208)*

304. **(A)** In placebo controlled trials, the agents that increase cAMP levels have adverse results, while agents that work by a different mechanism (digoxin) have a neutral effect on mortality. *(Katzung, p. 209)*

305. **(E)** Acute and chronic CHF are treated with different agents. Studies have indicated that the chronic use of agents that increase cAMP also increase mortality; these include beta-adrenergic agonists and phosphodiesterase inhibitors (methylxanthines, milrinone). Intravenous use of milrinone or dobutamine ($beta_1$ agonist) is effective acutely. *(Katzung, p. 209)*

306. **(E)** The first agents showing a decrease in mortality in chronic CHF were the combination of hydralazine and isosorbide dinitrate. However, this combination is now reserved for patients who are intolerant to ACE inhibitors since studies demonstrate the superiority of ACE inhibitor therapy over other treatments. *(Katzung, p. 213)*

307. **(C)** The cautious use of beta-adrenergic blocking agents is based on the concept that circulating catecholamines can cause fatal arrhythmias. This type of treatment protects the heart from those arrhythmias. In addition, carvedilol, which has $alpha_1$ blocking activity has been shown to reduce mortality. *(Katzung, p. 213)*

308. **(A)** Unless intoxication is severe, the correction of electrolyte levels coupled with monitoring of digoxin levels is usually sufficient to correct the problem within one to two half-lives (1 to 3 days). *(Katzung, p. 212)*

309. **(B)** In managing chronic CHF, ACE inhibitors are superior agents. However, patients already on digoxin will deteriorate if withdrawn from digoxin. Calcium channel blockers have no useful role. Aldosterone antagonists and angiotensin II receptor blockers are effective agents. *(Katzung, p. 213)*

310. **(D)** Digoxin has a half-life of 1½ days. Therefore, an initial dose is given to "digitalize" the patient. Digitoxin has a half-life of 7 days. These agents have very long half-lives compared with most pharmacologic agents. *(Katzung, p. 211)*

311. **(B)** Cardiac glycosides are widely distributed in plants and in certain toads. They do not require sugar residues for their action (it is found in the genin or aglycone) but do require an unsaturated lactone ring at position 17. They have steroid activity as evidenced by gynecomastia. *(Katzung, p. 204)*

312. **(E)** In addition to simvastatin, lovastatin is also administered in the inactive form and must be activated in the gut. All of the drugs have a half-life of approximately 1 to 3 hours except atorvastatin, $t_{1/2} = 14$ hours. *(Katzung, p. 591)*

313. **(B)** Low levels of HDL is an independent risk factor for coronary disease since these lipoproteins are active in removing cholesterol from the artery wall and in inhibiting oxidation of atherogenic lipoproteins. *(Katzung, p. 582)*

314. **(C)** The epidemiological data indicate that increased risk of coronary artery disease is associated with increased plasma lipoprotein levels. It is desirable to have total cholesterol levels below 200 mg/dL. *(Katzung, p. 584)*

315. **(C)** All of the conditions except early nephrosis will lead to elevated triglycerides. Early nephrosis leads to elevated cholesterol. These conditions should be treated prior to initiating treatment for primary hyperlipidemia. *(Katzung, pp. 585, 587)*

316. **(D)** Patients with premature atherosclerosis tend to have low HDL levels as the only identifiable risk factor. The most effective agent in increasing HDL levels is niacin. *(Katzung, p. 587)*

317. **(E)** The effects of dietary fats in patients with hypertriglyceridemias can be controlled by administering omega-3 fatty acids found in fish oils. Omega-6 fatty acids will increase triglycerides. Severe dietary restriction or lowering of homocysteine in the diet is most effective for elevated chylomicrons. Niacin and fibrates are more effective for hypertriglyceridemia than are the statins. *(Katzung, pp. 585–586)*

318. **(E)** Nitroglycerin has a short duration of action (minutes) and would be rapidly inactivated if given orally. *(Katzung, p. 184)*

319. **(C)** Isosorbide metabolites have longer half-lives (hours) making them orally effective agents. Amyl nitrite is administered by inhalation. Nitroglycerin and glyceryl trinitrate are administered sublingually. Nitric oxide is a gas. *(Katzung, p. 184)*

320. **(D)** The major body of evidence suggests that it is the reduction in oxygen requirement as a consequence of decreased preload that is primarily responsible for the effectiveness of nitroglycerin in angina pectoris. *(Katzung, p. 185)*

321. **(D)** The nitric oxide generated or the nitrites produced have very little direct effect on cardiac or skeletal muscle. *(Katzung, p. 185)*

322. **(A)** While the agents have been tried in all of the conditions listed, the short duration of action makes them clinically useless. Erectile dysfunction, however, has received a great deal of attention. The relaxation of smooth muscle results in increased blood flow to the penis. *(Katzung, pp. 185–186)*

323. **(A)** If an antihypertensive agent that is an effective arteriolar dilator is used, it is possible to shift blood away from a partially occluded vessel that is adequately perfusing the surrounding tissue when resistance is maintained. Lowering resistance in an adjacent vessel defers blood from the poorly perfused area and intensifies the angina. *(Katzung, p. 186)*

324. **(D)** Workers exposed to organic nitrates would rapidly develop tolerance to the compounds and rapidly lose the tolerance over the weekend. When they returned to work on Monday, the intense vasodilation resulted in headache. *(Katzung, p. 187)*

325. **(D)** Sildenafil, an inhibitor of phosphodiesterase isoform 5, causes the accumulation of cGMP and the generation of nitric oxide and allows blood to enter the penis, resulting in erection. Other than the use of PGE_1, analogs have not proven effective in clinical trials. *(Katzung, p. 187)*

326. **(C)** The primary relief of angina in angina of effort appears to be due to decreased myocardial oxygen consumption. In variant angina the effectiveness is based on relieving coronary artery spasm, and in unstable angina the major mechanism appears to be inhibition of platelet aggregation, thus inhibiting the formation of nonocclusive thrombi. *(Katzung, p. 188)*

327. **(B)** Diltiazem and verapamil belong to the miscellaneous group of agents. They do not affect skeletal muscle but have a greater effect on cardiac muscle than arteriolar or venous vascular smooth muscle. *(Katzung, pp. 191–192)*

328. **(C)** Some studies have reported limiting infarct size by preventing calcium entry. All of the other statements are exactly the opposite of the statement: Insulin release is inhibited;

morbidity in subarachnoid hemorrhage is decreased; short-acting agents have a high negative inotropic effect; and, due to different types of receptors, these agents have little effect on stimulus secretion coupling. *(Katzung, pp. 191–192)*

329. **(E)** Due to the fact that it is more selective for the heart, the most appropriate agent would be verapamil. *(Katzung, pp. 193–194)*

330. **(B)** While redistribution of blood flow may occur, the objective is to decrease oxygen demand. Reducing heart rate, blood pressure, and contractile force development is a major effect of beta blockers and will definitely lead to a decrease in oxygen demand. Beta-adrenergic blocking agents are not vasodilators. *(Katzung, pp. 194–195)*

331. **(B)** The most effective approach would be to add another class of agents—in this case, calcium channel blocker, or if the choice were given, a nitrate could be selected. Increasing the propranolol will probably increase the feeling of being tired, and another drug from the same class, metoprolol, may not be any more effective. Adding two additional classes of agents is premature. Changing his profession might be a suggestion, but it will probably not be acceptable to him. *(Katzung, p. 196)*

332. **(E)** Warfarin produces its anticoagulant effect by interfering with the vitamin K–dependent gamma-carboxylation of glutamate residues in the vitamin K–dependent clotting factors. Administration of vitamin K to the patient can overcome this effect of warfarin. *(Katzung, p. 572)*

333. **(E)** Rifampin induces the enzymes that transform racemic warfarin in the body. Whereas metronidazole and fluconazole inhibit biotransformation of S-warfarin, amiodarone and cimetidine inhibit the biotransformation of both enantiomorphs. *(Katzung, pp. 571–572)*

334. **(A)** Aminocaproic acid is a synthetic compound that is chemically similar to lysine and is a competitive inhibitor of plasminogen activation. *(Katzung, p. 578)*

335. **(D)** Lepirudin is the recombinant form of hirudin, a specific thrombin inhibitor from the leech. *(Katzung, p. 569)*

336. **(C)** Patients with reduced kidney functions should not be given carbonic anhydrase inhibitors or potassium-sparing diuretics, and thiazides are usually ineffective if the glomerular filtration rate (GFR) is low. The loop diuretics are the best choice. *(Katzung, pp. 260–261)*

337. **(B)** Osmotic diuretics act at sites where the nephron is freely permeable to water. The compound is not absorbed; it remains in the nephron after filtration and creates osmotic pressure, holding water in the nephron. This action results in a reduction of total body water and results in a reduction of intracranial pressure. *(Katzung, p. 258)*

338. **(C)** Loop diuretics act at the site of calcium reabsorption, thus preventing resorption and promoting calcium diuresis. However, it is necessary to administer saline simultaneously since contraction of fluid volume can accentuate the hypercalcemia. *(Katzung, p. 262)*

339. **(D)** The thiazides still play an important role in patients who require multiple drugs to control blood pressure; they enhance the efficacy of ACE inhibitors and prevent volume retention in patients treated with vasodilators. These agents are also important because of their low cost. *(Katzung, p. 262)*

340. **(F)** Aldosterone antagonists (spironolactone) effectively counteract the high levels of aldosterone often found in these patients. *(Katzung, p. 261)*

341. **(A)** Carbonic anhydrase inhibition leads to depletion in the body bicarbonate stores. However, since bicarbonate can be reabsorbed by noncarbonic anhydrase-dependent sites, it loses its effectiveness. Acetazolamide, the prototype, is rarely used for diuresis but is used to reduce production of aqueous humor or cerebral spinal fluid. *(Katzung, pp. 251–252)*

342. **(C)** The action of thiazides, loop diuretics, spironolactone, and triamterene are all dependent on renal prostaglandin production. *(Katzung, pp. 255, 257)*

343. **(D)** Technically, diuresis refers to an increase in urine volume. The term *natriuresis* indicates a loss of sodium ion, while *kaluresis* is a loss of potassium ion. *(Katzung, p. 245)*

344. **(B)** The loop diuretics cause a dose-related loss of hearing that is usually reversible. They should be avoided in patients with hearing loss or in patients who are on other ototoxic drugs such as gentamicin or aminoglycoside antibiotics. *(Katzung, p. 254)*

345. **(B)** ADH inhibits aldosterone receptors located in the cortical collecting duct and late distal tubule. Aldosterone promotes retention of sodium and enhances potassium secretion. Sodium absorption leads to potassium loss to balance the electrical gradient. Aldosterone antagonists reduce potassium loss (potassium sparing) by inhibiting aldosterone action. *(Katzung, pp. 256–257)*

346. **(A)** The adherence to a low-sodium diet may prevent the development of hypokalemia. High sodium leads to increased potassium secretion. Hypokalemia in the presence of digoxin would be expected to cause arrhythmias. Administration of potassium is not routinely necessary. *(Katzung, p. 260)*

347. **(E)** The aldosterone antagonists may cause severe hyperkalemia in the presence of altered renal function, agents that inhibit renin formation (beta blockers), or agents that reduce angiotensin II activity (ACE inhibitors, angiotensin receptor blockers). *(Katzung, p. 257)*

348. **(E)** Compounds that inhibit aldosterone, synthetic steroids, may cause gynecomastia, BPH, impotence, or other endocrine abnormalities. *(Katzung, p. 257)*

349. **(D)** ACE converts angiotensin I to angiotensin II and also converts bradykinin to

an inactive compound. Inhibiting ACE results in increased bradykinin levels. This increase is postulated to be the cause of ACE-induced cough. *(Katzung, pp. 173–174)*

350. **(F)** African Americans respond to agents (diuretics) that lower sodium ion and thus reduce vascular volume. Calcium channel blockers are effective in this group of patients. Either of these agents is more effective than beta blockers or ACE inhibitors. *(Katzung, p. 175)*

351. **(J)** The most accepted theory explaining the hypotensive action of clonidine is based on stimulation of alpha$_2$-adrenergic receptors in the vasomotor center. This stimulation results in a decrease in sympathetic outflow. *(Katzung, p. 161)*

352. **(B)** The blockade of beta-adrenergic receptors on the juxtaglomerular cells of the kidney is thought to be responsible for the hypotensive action of beta receptor blockers. *(Katzung, p. 166)*

353. **(H)** Both of these agents cause depletion of norepinephrine in the adrenergic nerve endings, resulting in prevention of the physiologic release of this pressor agent. *(Katzung, pp. 163–165)*

354. **(C)** The administration of nonselective alpha-blocking agents inhibits vascular tone by blocking peripheral alpha$_1$ receptors, but these compounds also block alpha$_2$ receptors in the myocardium. Blocking these receptors results in increased release of norepinephrine and tachycardia due to beta$_1$ receptor stimulation. This is the rationale for using selective beta$_1$ agents. *(Katzung, p. 168)*

355. **(F)** With the exception of spironolactone, this is a true statement. Both the thiazides and the loop diuretics may result in symptomatic potassium loss. *(Katzung, p. 159)*

356. **(C)** Both carvedilol and labetalol nonselectively block beta receptors. They also decrease peripheral resistance by blocking alpha$_1$ receptors. *(Katzung, p. 167)*

357. **(D)** Quinidine is considered an Ia agent. The class I agents are sodium channel blockers and are further classified by their effect on the duration of the action potential. Ia lengthens the duration; Ib shortens the duration; Ic has minimal effect on the duration. *(Katzung, pp. 229–230)*

358. **(B)** Local anesthetics are sodium channel blockers. Lidocaine is a widely used local anesthetic that is administered intravenously to suppress arrhythmias. *(Katzung, p. 229)*

359. **(C)** Metoprolol is easily identified as a beta-adrenergic blocking agent by its "-olol" ending. It inhibits the development of arrhythmias due to increased excitability when increased amounts of norepinephrine are released or when circulating levels of epinephrine are elevated. *(Katzung, p. 229)*

360. **(A)** Amiodarone is a potassium channel blocker that prolongs the duration of the action potential by blocking outward or augmenting inward currents. *(Katzung, p. 234)*

361. **(E)** Calcium channel blockers of the nondihydropyridine type are effective in inhibiting cardiac calcium currents in the AV node and thus protecting the ventricle from aberrant electrical activity in the atrial muscle. *(Katzung, p. 239)*

362. **(B)** Hypertriglyceridemias in which VLDL predominates are most effectively treated with the fibrates. *(Katzung, p. 590)*

363. **(A)** Cholesterol is metabolized to bile acids and reabsorbed with high efficiency (95%) from the jejunum and ileum. The administration of resins results in excretion of these bile acids before they can be reabsorbed. *(Katzung, p. 590)*

364. **(A)** The bile acid–binding resins will impair the absorption of numerous pharmacologic agents, including tetracyclines, iron salts, the statins, folic acid, aspirin, the thiazides, and others as well as those indicated in the question. *(Katzung, p. 591)*

365. **(D)** The so-called "statins" inhibit the enzyme HMG-CoA reductase, which mediates the first committed step in sterol biosynthesis. *(Katzung, p. 591)*

366. **(C)** Niacin (not nicotinamide) causes a harmless cutaneous vasodilation that appears to be prostaglandin mediated. NSAIDs blunt the response. This, along with pruritus, rashes, and dry skin, is not well accepted by patients. *(Katzung, p. 589)*

367. **(D)** The statins may cause an elevation of creatine kinase levels associated with a skeletal muscle myopathy. Patients who experience muscle pain, soreness, or weakness should have the statin discontinued immediately. Rechallenge with another statin remains a possibility. *(Katzung, p. 593)*

368. **(C)** In familial hypercholesteremia, the combination of a reductase inhibitor and niacin appears to be better than either agent alone. *(Katzung, p. 586)*

369. **(D)** ET-I initially releases prostacyclin and nitric oxide from the endothelium and then directly contracts vascular smooth muscle. It is a mitogen, and it also causes constriction of airway smooth muscle. Agents that block the action of this peptide are being explored for use in pulmonary hypertension and chronic heart failure. *(Katzung, pp. 303–305)*

370. **(B)** ANP is a natriuretic, diuretic, and vasorelaxant peptide. Patients with heart failure have elevated ANP in their plasma, an indication that they act to reduce salt and water retention. *(Katzung, pp. 302–303)*

371. **(C)** Bradykinin causes vasodilation directly or through the release of nitric oxide or PGE_2. The vasoconstriction is due to direct contraction of venous smooth muscle or to release of PGF_2. ANP is 10 times more potent than histamine. *(Katzung, p. 299)*

372. **(A)** Angiotensinogen is converted to angiotensin I and then to angiotensin II. Angiotensin II is 40 times more potent than nor-

epinephrine in increasing blood pressure. It also stimulates the release of aldosterone. *(Katzung, pp. 293–294)*

373. **(G)** Vasopressin is also known as antidiuretic hormone. In addition to its role in retaining water, it has a vasoconstrictor action. *(Katzung, p. 301)*

374. **(F)** This peptide does not act through adrenergic, cholinergic, histaminergic, or serotonergic receptors. It may be released from nonadrenergic, noncholinergic (NANC) fibers. *(Katzung, pp. 305–306)*

375. **(F)** Fibrinogen, vitronectin, fibronectin, and von Willebrand factor can bind to the IIb/IIIa receptor complex and thereby mediate platelet aggregation by anchoring platelets to foreign surfaces and to each other. Abciximab is a monoclonal antibody that binds to and blocks the platelet IIb/IIIa receptor complex. *(Katzung, p. 575)*

376. **(E)** Thromboxane A_2 promotes platelet degranulation and aggregation. By blocking the synthesis of this arachidonate product, aspirin interferes with platelet function. *(Katzung, p. 574)*

377. **(G)** ADP is released from platelets by thrombin and is an inducer of platelet aggregation. By blocking the binding of ADP to its receptor, clopidogrel reduces platelet aggregation. *(Katzung, pp. 564, 574–575)*

378. **(F)** Fibrinogen, vitronectin, fibronectin, and von Willebrand factor can bind to the IIb/IIIa receptor complex and thereby mediate platelet aggregation by anchoring platelets to foreign surfaces and to each other. Eptifibatide is an analog of the portion of the fibrinogen molecule that binds to the IIb/IIIa receptor complex. *(Katzung, p. 575; Hardman et al., p. 1535)*

379. **(D)** Low-molecular-weight heparins (e.g., enoxaparin and dalteparin) have less effect on antithrombin and coagulation in general

than unfractionated heparin, which acts mainly by mechanisms utilizing antithrombin III as a cofactor. *(Katzung, pp. 567–568)*

380. **(C)** Activated plasmin affects the dissolution of the thrombus by proteolytic digestion of fibrin. *(Katzung, pp 565–566, 572–574)*

381. **(F)** Tirofiban contains the main amino acid recognition sequence for the platelet IIb/IIIa receptor complex. *(Katzung, p. 575)*

382. **(A)** Because overdose with unfractionated heparin can lead to bleeding and too low a dose can result in inadequate protection of the patient from thrombus formation, it is essential to monitor the effect of this agent and adjust the dosage to achieve the proper degree of anticoagulation. The aPTT is the assay generally used for this purpose. *(Katzung, pp. 567–568)*

383. **(B)** Warfarin interferes with the ability of vitamin K to promote the carboxylation of glutamate residues on vitamin K–dependent clotting factors, thereby rendering these clotting factors incapable of participating in the clotting process. *(Katzung, p. 570)*

CHAPTER 5

Drugs Affecting Metabolic and Endocrine Function
Questions

DIRECTIONS (Questions 384 through 461): Each of the numbered items or incomplete statements in this section is followed by answers or by completions of the statement. Select the ONE lettered answer or completion that is BEST in each case.

384. Which of the following is the most common cause of chronic anemia?

    (A) folic acid deficiency
    (B) hematopoietic growth factor deficiency
    (C) iron deficiency
    (D) vitamin B_{12} deficiency
    (E) none of the above

385. Which of the following forms of iron is (are) appropriate for parenteral administration?

    (A) ferrous fumarate
    (B) ferrous gluconate
    (C) ferrous sulfate
    (D) iron dextran
    (E) all of the above

386. Which of the following statements is NOT true concerning vitamin B_{12} deficiency?

    (A) It typically results in megaloblastic anemia.
    (B) The anemia can be corrected by administration cyanocobalamin.
    (C) The anemia can be corrected by administration of folic acid.
    (D) The neurologic manifestations can be prevented by administration of cyanocobalamin.

    (E) The neurologic manifestations can be prevented by administration of folic acid.

387. Which of the following pharmacologic agents is most likely to be effective treatment for pernicious anemia?

    (A) erythropoietin
    (B) ferrous sulfate
    (C) folic acid
    (D) hydroxocobalamin
    (E) iron dextran

388. Which of the following pharmacologic agents would be best to treat the anemia caused by chronic renal failure?

    (A) erythropoietin
    (B) ferrous sulfate
    (C) folic acid
    (D) hydroxocobalamin
    (E) iron dextran

389. Which of the following conditions will likely respond to granulocyte colony-stimulating factor (G-CSF)?

    (A) anemia associated with chronic renal failure
    (B) microcytic hypochromic anemia
    (C) neutropenia caused by cancer chemotherapy
    (D) thrombocytopenia caused by cancer chemotherapy
    (E) all of the above

390. Which of the following substances provides a cofactor that is required for the one-carbon transfer reaction needed for production of deoxythymidylate (dTMP)?

    (A) folic acid
    (B) transferrin
    (C) vitamin D
    (D) vitamin K
    (E) all of the above

391. 11-*cis*-Retinal is a component of which of the following biologically active molecules?

    (A) menaquinone
    (B) opsin
    (C) phytonadione
    (D) rhodopsin
    (E) all of the above

392. Symptoms of hypervitaminosis A include which of the following?

    (A) erythematous dermatitis
    (B) neurologic symptoms
    (C) pain and tenderness of bones
    (D) papilledema
    (E) all of the above

393. Which of the following pharmacologic agents is used to prevent hypoprothrombinemia of the newborn?

    (A) folic acid
    (B) vitamin A
    (C) vitamin B_1
    (D) vitamin B_{12}
    (E) vitamin K_1

394. Which of the following pharmacologic agents may be useful in treating hypocalcemia associated with chronic renal failure?

    (A) calcitonin
    (B) etidronate
    (C) parathyroid hormone (PTH)
    (D) vitamin D
    (E) all of the above

395. Elevation of which of the following substances in the serum is diagnostic of hypervitaminosis D?

    (A) 1,25-dihydroxyvitamin D
    (B) 1-hydroxyvitamin D
    (C) 25-hydroxyvitamin D
    (D) calcium
    (E) PTH

396. Which step(s) in the conversion of vitamin D_3 to calcitriol is (are) carried out in the kidney?

    (A) hydroxylation of both the 1 and 25 carbons
    (B) hydroxylation of both the 3 and 25 carbons
    (C) hydroxylation of the 1 carbon only
    (D) hydroxylation of the 25 carbon only
    (E) hydroxylation of the 3 carbon only

397. What are the effects of PTH on the kidney?

    (A) decreased excretion of both calcium and phosphate
    (B) decreased excretion of calcium, but increased excretion of phosphate
    (C) increased excretion of both calcium and phosphate
    (D) increased excretion of calcium, but decreased excretion of phosphate
    (E) no effect on the excretion of calcium or phosphate

398. What is the effect of calcitriol (1,25-dihydroxyvitamin D) on the absorption of calcium and phosphate from bone and intestine?

    (A) decreased calcium and phosphate absorption from bone, increased absorption of both calcium and phosphate from the intestine
    (B) decreased calcium and phosphate absorption from bone, increased absorption of calcium and decreased absorption of phosphate from the intestine
    (C) increased calcium and phosphate absorption from bone, decreased absorption of both calcium and phosphate from the intestine

(D) increased calcium and phosphate absorption from bone, increased absorption of both calcium and phosphate from the intestine

(E) increased calcium and phosphate absorption from bone, increased absorption of calcium and decreased absorption of phosphate from the intestine

399. What is the principal toxicity of etidronate that is not seen with alendronate when high doses are used such as in treatment of Paget's disease?

(A) kidney damage
(B) liver toxicity
(C) muscle weakness
(D) neurologic symptoms
(E) osteomalacia

400. Which of the following drugs would be expected to help increase bone density in a patient with osteoporosis?

(A) alendronate
(B) dexamethasone
(C) PTH
(D) triamcinolone
(E) all of the above

401. Which of the following agents has (have) proved useful for treating cases of hypercalcemia?

(A) calcitonin
(B) etidronate
(C) furosemide
(D) gallium nitrate
(E) all of the above

402. Which of the following is the major mechanism of the contractile action of oxytocin on the pregnant uterus?

(A) activation of receptors coupled to a G-protein (G_q), which activates the calcium–phosphoinositide-signaling pathway

(B) activation of intracellular receptors that regulate transcription of selected genes

(C) activation of receptors coupled directly to sodium channels on the cell membrane

(D) activation of receptors coupled directly to tyrosine kinase

(E) activation of receptors coupled to a G-protein (G_s), which activates the adenylyl cyclase/cyclic adenosine monophosphate (cAMP) signaling pathway

403. Which of the following adverse effects has (have) resulted from the overadministration of oxytocin to pregnant mothers?

(A) fetal deaths due to compromised fetal oxygenation
(B) maternal deaths due to hypertensive episodes
(C) uterine rupture
(D) water intoxication
(E) all of the above

404. What type of administration of gonadotropin-releasing hormone (GnRH) would be most suitable for promoting fertility in women?

(A) intramuscular (IM) injection
(B) intranasal administration by spray
(C) intravenous (IV) administration in pulses
(D) oral administration
(E) transdermal administration by a patch

405. Leuprolide is a synthetic chemical analog of which of the following naturally occurring hormones?

(A) estradiol
(B) follicle-stimulating hormone (FSH)
(C) GnRH
(D) luteinizing hormone (LH)
(E) progesterone

406. A woman being treated with gonadotropins to promote fertility develops abdominal pain and distention, nausea and vomiting, diarrhea, dyspnea, and oliguria. These symptoms are most likely caused by the direct effect of the gonadotropins on which of the following organ systems?

    (A) gastrointestinal (GI) tract
    (B) heart
    (C) kidney
    (D) liver
    (E) ovary

407. Implantation of a depot preparation of leuprolide can result in which of the following long-term effects?

    (A) long-term inhibition of gonadotropin release from the pituitary gland
    (B) long-term stimulation of estrogen production in the ovary
    (C) long-term stimulation of gonadotropin release from the pituitary gland
    (D) long-term stimulation of progesterone production in the ovary
    (E) none of the above

408. What is the correct order of potency of the following compounds: 3,5,3'-triiodothyronine (T_3), 3,3',5'-triiodothyronine (reverse T_3) and thyroxine (T_4)?

    (A) T_3 > reverse T_3 > T_4
    (B) reverse T_3 > T_3 > T_4
    (C) T_4 > T_3 > reverse T_3
    (D) T_3 > T_4 > reverse T_3
    (E) reverse T_3 > T_4 > T_3

409. What percentage of circulating thyroid hormones is free (not bound by plasma proteins)?

    (A) < 1%
    (B) 5 to 10%
    (C) 20 to 30%
    (D) 40 to 50%
    (E) > 50%

410. Which of the following factors influence(s) the absorption of orally administered levothyroxine?

    (A) aluminum-containing antacids
    (B) food
    (C) iron
    (D) sucralfate
    (E) all of the above

411. Which of the following best describes the main mechanism of action of thyroid hormones?

    (A) They activate receptors in the cell nucleus, modulating the formation of messenger RNA (mRNA) coding for certain proteins.
    (B) They activate receptors on cell membranes coupled to G-proteins.
    (C) They activate receptors on cell membranes, resulting in the activation of intracellular tyrosine kinase.
    (D) They activate receptors on cell membranes, resulting in the opening of sodium channels.
    (E) They bind directly to nuclear DNA, thereby impeding gene transcription.

412. The use of phenytoin by a hypothyroid patient being treated with thyroxine would most likely result in which of the following effects?

    (A) decreased metabolism of T_4 due to inhibition of hepatic enzyme activity
    (B) displacement of T_4 from binding sites on thyroxine-binding globulin (TBG)
    (C) increased metabolism of T_4 due to induction of increased hepatic enzyme activity
    (D) interference with levothyroxine absorption from the GI tract
    (E) none of the above

413. Which thyroid hormone preparation is the agent of choice for thyroid replacement therapy?

    (A) levothyroxine (T_4)
    (B) liothyronine (T_3)
    (C) liotrix ($T_4 + T_3$)
    (D) thyroid desiccated (USP)
    (E) none of the above

414. Methimazole and propylthiouracil belong to which class of drugs?

    (A) benzodiazepines
    (B) methylxanthines
    (C) organophosphates
    (D) sulfonamides
    (E) thioamides

415. What is the main reason methimazole can be given only once a day for management of mild to moderate hyperthyroidism?

    (A) It is accumulated by the thyroid gland.
    (B) It is metabolized to active metabolites.
    (C) It is very tightly bound by plasma proteins.
    (D) Its half-life in the plasma is 12 hours.
    (E) none of the above

416. Which of the following mechanisms is (are) thought to be involved in producing the antithyroid action of propylthiouracil?

    (A) inhibition of peroxidase-catalyzed reactions to block iodine organification in the thyroid gland
    (B) inhibition of the release of thyroid hormones from the thyroid gland
    (C) inhibition of the uptake of iodide into the thyroid gland
    (D) all of the above
    (E) none of the above

417. In general, how fast is the onset of the antithyroid action of methimazole?

    (A) < 2 hours
    (B) 3 to 4 hours
    (C) 3 to 4 days
    (D) 3 to 4 weeks
    (E) 3 to 4 months

418. Which of the following pharmacologic agents increase(s) the binding of thyroxine by TBG?

    (A) androgens
    (B) estrogens
    (C) furosemide
    (D) glucocorticoids
    (E) salicylates

419. What is the major mechanism of the antithyroid action of potassium perchlorate?

    (A) blockade of the coupling of iodotyrosines in the thyroid gland
    (B) competitive inhibition of the uptake of iodide into the thyroid gland
    (C) inhibition of peroxidase-catalyzed reactions, resulting in blockade of iodine organification in the thyroid gland
    (D) inhibition of the peripheral deiodination of T_4 and T_3
    (E) inhibition of the release of preformed thyroid hormones from the thyroid gland

420. What is (are) the major mechanism(s) of the antithyroid action of pharmacologic doses of iodide?

    (A) blockade of the coupling of iodotyrosines in the thyroid gland
    (B) competitive inhibition of the uptake of iodide into the thyroid gland
    (C) inhibition of the peripheral deiodination of T_4 and T_3
    (D) inhibition of the release of preformed thyroid hormones from the thyroid gland
    (E) all of the above

421. What is the major mechanism of action of glucocorticoids?

    (A) They activate receptors on cell membranes coupled to G-proteins that activate the phosphoinositide-signaling pathway.
    (B) They activate receptors on cell membranes coupled to G-proteins that activate the cAMP-signaling pathway.
    (C) They activate receptors on cell membranes resulting in the activation of intracellular tyrosine kinase.
    (D) They bind to receptors in the cytoplasm that translocate to the nucleus, where they regulate the transcription of certain genes.
    (E) They activate receptors on cell membranes, resulting in the opening of sodium channels.

422. Which of the following hormones produce(s) a lipolytic response that is attenuated in the absence of glucocorticoids?

    (A) adrenocorticotropic hormone (ACTH)
    (B) catecholamines
    (C) growth hormone
    (D) all of the above
    (E) none of the above

423. Which of the following is (are) a major effect(s) of glucocorticoids on vascular and airway smooth muscle?

    (A) increase in the tone of these smooth muscles
    (B) increased responsiveness of these tissues to the metabolic effects of insulin
    (C) increased responsiveness of these tissues to the relaxant effects of catecholamines
    (D) all of the above
    (E) none of the above

424. Which of the following factors contribute(s) to the lipogenesis that occurs after administration of glucocorticoids to a patient?

    (A) the direct effect of glucocorticoids on lipoprotein lipase

    (B) the "permissive effect" of glucocorticoids on the responsiveness of adipose tissues to ACTH
    (C) the release of insulin from the pancreas
    (D) all of the above
    (E) none of the above

425. Although glucocorticoids stimulate protein and RNA synthesis in the liver, they have a catabolic effect on which of the following tissues?

    (A) bone
    (B) lymphoid and connective tissue
    (C) skeletal muscle
    (D) skin
    (E) all of the above

426. Which type of leukocyte increases in concentration in the blood after a single dose of short-acting glucocorticoid?

    (A) basophils
    (B) eosinophils
    (C) lymphocytes
    (D) monocytes
    (E) neutrophils

427. Which of the following functions of tissue macrophages is (are) reduced by glucocorticoids?

    (A) ability to phagocytose and kill microorganisms
    (B) ability to produce interleukin-12 and interferon-gamma
    (C) ability to produce tumor necrosis factor-alpha, interleukin-1, metalloproteinases, and plasminogen activator
    (D) ability to respond to antigens and mitogens
    (E) all of the above

428. Glucocorticoids are most likely to interfere with the action of which of the following vitamins?

    (A) vitamin A
    (B) vitamin C
    (C) vitamin D

(D) vitamin E

(E) vitamin K

429. Which of the following synthetic steroids has the greatest relative salt-retaining activity?

(A) betamethasone

(B) dexamethasone

(C) fludrocortisone

(D) fluprednisolone

(E) prednisone

430. Which of the following steroids has the longest duration of action?

(A) cortisone

(B) dexamethasone

(C) prednisolone

(D) prednisone

(E) triamcinolone

431. Which of the following pharmacologic agents is most often administered to pregnant mothers to prevent the incidence of respiratory distress syndrome in infants delivered prematurely?

(A) betamethasone

(B) desoxycorticosterone acetate

(C) fludrocortisone

(D) levothyroxine

(E) vitamin C

432. Which of the following corticosteroids, when administered in pharmacologic doses, is most likely to cause sodium and fluid retention and loss of potassium?

(A) betamethasone

(B) dexamethasone

(C) hydrocortisone

(D) methylprednisolone

(E) triamcinolone

433. Which of the following conditions is LEAST likely to occur in response to administration of glucocorticoids for longer than 2 weeks?

(A) elevation of blood glucose levels

(B) increased appetite

(C) insomnia

(D) redistribution of fat from the extremities to the trunk

(E) thin, emaciated facial features

434. Which of the following is (are) a known complication(s) of long-term glucocorticoid therapy?

(A) muscle wasting

(B) osteoporosis

(C) peptic ulcers

(D) thinning of the skin

(E) all of the above

435. Estrogens are known to stimulate the synthesis of which of the following types of receptors?

(A) estrogen receptors

(B) FSH receptors

(C) GnRH receptors

(D) LH receptors

(E) progesterone receptors

436. Administration of estrogens to estrogen-deficient female patients is LEAST likely to produce which of the following?

(A) fertility

(B) secondary sex characteristics

(C) prevention of osteoporosis

(D) growth of the uterus

(E) optimal body growth

437. What is the main reason for including a progestin in hormonal replacement therapy in postmenopausal women?

(A) to increase plasma concentrations of high-density lipoprotein (HDL)

(B) to lower plasma concentrations of low-density lipoprotein (LDL)

(C) to reduce the risk of breast cancer

(D) to reduce the risk of endometrial cancer

(E) all of the above

438. Which of the following are effects produced by hormone replacement therapy in postmenopausal women?

(A) reduction of the risk of osteoporosis
(B) relief of atropic vaginitis
(C) relief of hot flashes
(D) relief of excessive sweating
(E) all of the above

439. Which of the following is (are) a risk factor(s) for osteoporosis?

(A) being Caucasian
(B) inactive lifestyle
(C) smoking
(D) strong family history of osteoporosis
(E) all of the above

440. Currently prescribed doses of estrogens in hormone replacement therapy are LEAST likely to increase the frequency or risk of which of the following adverse conditions?

(A) breast tenderness
(B) gallbladder disease
(C) hypertension
(D) migraine headaches
(E) venous thromboembolism

441. Progesterone or other progestins are LEAST likely to produce which of the following effects?

(A) alteration of endocervical secretions from an abundant watery product to a scant, viscid material
(B) development of a secretory endometrium
(C) enhancement of estrogen-driven endometrial proliferation
(D) suppression of menstruation during pregnancy
(E) suppression of uterine contraction during pregnancy

442. Which of the following adverse effects is most common with the continuous use of a progestin alone to prevent pregnancy?

(A) acne
(B) breakthrough bleeding
(C) decreased glucose tolerance
(D) hypertension
(E) weight gain

443. Which of the following statements about venous thromboembolic disease associated with the use of combination oral contraceptives is (are) correct?

(A) The incidence of this disorder is related to the estrogen but not the progestin content of the oral contraceptive.
(B) The increased risk of venous thromboembolism lasts for about 3 years after use of oral contraceptives is stopped.
(C) The overall incidence of venous thromboembolism in women taking low-dose oral contraceptives is about 15-fold higher than in women not taking contraceptives.
(D) This adverse effect is associated with an increase in plasma antithrombin III levels.
(E) all of the above

444. Which of the following represents the most likely adverse response to androgenic/anabolic steroids used to stimulate growth in boys with delayed puberty?

(A) aplastic anemia
(B) arrest of growth before reaching full final stature
(C) decreased bone mineral density
(D) muscle wasting and weakness
(E) thinning of the skin with bruising and striae

445. Use of anabolic/androgenic steroids is contraindicated in which of the following conditions?

(A) acquired immune deficiency syndrome (AIDS)
(B) angioneurotic edema
(C) aplastic anemia

(D) carcinoma of the prostate gland

(E) osteoporosis

446. The principal side effects of the 17α-alkylated androgens are on which of the following organ systems?

(A) autonomic nervous system

(B) heart

(C) kidneys

(D) liver

(E) skeletal muscle

447. What is the half-life of circulating insulin?

(A) 3 to 5 minutes

(B) 35 to 40 minutes

(C) 3 to 5 hours

(D) 8 to 10 hours

(E) 18 to 24 hours

448. Which of the following statements about the effects of insulin on the liver is most accurate?

(A) It inhibits the conversion of amino acids to glucose.

(B) It inhibits triglyceride synthesis.

(C) It inhibits very-low-density lipoprotein (VLDL) formation.

(D) It stimulates glycogenolysis.

(E) It stimulates the conversion of fatty acids to keto acids.

449. Which of the following insulin preparations has the longest duration of action?

(A) insulin lispro

(B) Lente insulin

(C) NPH (neutral protamine Hagedorn) insulin

(D) regular insulin

(E) Ultralente insulin

450. Which of the following conditions is the most common complication of insulin therapy?

(A) diabetes insipidus

(B) hypertension

(C) hypoglycemia

(D) orthostatic hypotension

(E) retinal degeneration

451. Which of the following represents the main mechanism of action of sulfonylurea antidiabetic drugs?

(A) They act as agonists for nuclear peroxisome proliferator-activated receptor gamma (PPARγ), which activates insulin-responsive genes.

(B) They have a direct effect on liver enzymes to inhibit gluconeogenesis.

(C) They have a direct effect on liver enzymes to promote glycogen storage.

(D) They inhibit the efflux of potassium ions through adenosine triphosphate (ATP)-sensitive potassium channels in pancreatic B-cell membranes.

(E) They inhibit alpha-glucosidase activity in the intestine.

452. Which of the following represents the main mechanism of action of thiazolidinedione antidiabetic drugs?

(A) They act as agonists for nuclear PPARγ, which activates insulin-responsive genes.

(B) They have a direct effect on liver enzymes to inhibit gluconeogenesis.

(C) They have a direct effect on liver enzymes to promote glycogen storage.

(D) They inhibit the efflux of potassium ions through ATP-sensitive potassium channels in pancreatic B-cell membranes.

(E) They inhibit alpha-glucosidase activity in the intestine.

453. Which of the following represents the main mechanism of the antidiabetic action of acarbose and miglitol?

(A) They act as agonists for nuclear PPARγ, which activates insulin-responsive genes.

(B) They have a direct effect on liver enzymes to inhibit gluconeogenesis.

(C) They have a direct effect on liver enzymes to promote glycogen storage.

(D) They inhibit the efflux of potassium ions through ATP-sensitive potassium channels in pancreatic B-cell membranes.

(E) They inhibit α-glucosidase activity in the intestine.

454. Which of the following represents the main mechanism of action of repaglinide and nateglinide?

(A) They act principally to lower insulin resistance in peripheral tissues.

(B) They act principally to release insulin from the pancreas.

(C) They have a direct effect on liver enzymes to inhibit gluconeogenesis.

(D) They have a direct effect on liver enzymes to promote glycogen storage.

(E) They slow the absorption of carbohydrates from the intestine.

455. Glyburide, glimepiride, and glipizide are members of which group of drugs?

(A) biguanides

(B) first-generation sulfonylureas

(C) meglitinides

(D) second-generation sulfonylureas

(E) thiazolidinediones

456. Rosiglitazone and pioglitazone are members of which group of drugs?

(A) biguanides

(B) first-generation sulfonylureas

(C) meglitinides

(D) second-generation sulfonylureas

(E) thiazolidinediones

457. Which of the following conditions represent(s) the most common toxic reaction(s) to glyburide when used as a single antidiabetic agent?

(A) gastrointestinal (GI) disturbances

(B) hypertension

(C) hypoglycemia

(D) interference with calcium absorption from the GI tract

(E) orthostatic hypotension

458. Which of the following is a relatively new insulin secretagogue with a very rapid onset and short duration of action that make it especially suitable for controlling postprandial glucose excursions?

(A) glimepiride

(B) glyburide

(C) metformin

(D) pioglitazone

(E) repaglinide

459. What is (are) the most common adverse reaction(s) to alpha-glucosidase inhibitors?

(A) central nervous system (CNS) disturbances

(B) GI disturbances

(C) hypertension

(D) hypoglycemia

(E) liver toxicity

460. Which of the following can precipitate symptoms of thiamine deficiency in marginally nourished patients?

(A) glucose

(B) riboflavin

(C) thiazide diuretics

(D) vitamin B_{12}

(E) vitamin E

461. Which of the following vitamins can be used for prophylaxis and treatment of pellagra?

(A) biotin

(B) inositol

(C) nicotinic acid

(D) pantothenic acid

(E) riboflavin

Answers and Explanations

384. (C) Iron deficiency is the most common cause of chronic anemia. The absence of adequate amounts of iron gives rise to microcytic hypochromic anemia in which small erythrocytes with insufficient amounts of hemoglobin are formed. This form of anemia can usually be treated effectively with preparations of ferrous sulfate, ferrous gluconate, or ferrous fumarate for oral administration. *(Katzung, pp. 549, 551)*

385. (D) Iron dextran is a stable complex of ferric hydroxide and low-molecular-weight dextran, which can be given either by IM injection or IV infusion. *(Katzung, pp. 551–552)*

386. (E) Although folic acid will largely correct the anemia caused by vitamin B_{12} deficiency, it will not prevent the potentially irreversible neurologic manifestations. *(Katzung, pp. 552–554)*

387. (D) Pernicious anemia is caused by malabsorption of vitamin B_{12} from the intestine, usually because of the failure of gastric mucosae to secrete intrinsic factor, which is required for absorption of the vitamin. Parenteral administration of hydroxocobalamin (vitamin B_{12}) can be used to treat this condition. *(Katzung, pp. 554–555)*

388. (A) Chronic renal failure can result in a decreased output of erythropoietin, leading to a low hematocrit and hemoglobin. Recombinant erythropoietin can increase the hematocrit and hemoglobin in these patients. *(Katzung, pp. 558–559)*

389. (C) Recombinant G-CSF can accelerate the rate of neutrophil recovery after myelosuppressive chemotherapy. It does not stimulate the production of erythrocytes or platelets. *(Katzung, pp. 559–561)*

390. (A) Tetrahydrofolate cofactors participate in one-carbon transfer reactions, one of which is essential for the production of dTMP, needed for DNA synthesis. *(Katzung, pp. 553–557)*

391. (D) 11-*cis*-Retinal is a member of the vitamin A family and combines with opsin to form rhodopsin, the holoreceptor in retinal rods. *(Hardman et al., pp. 1773–1776)*

392. (E) Symptoms of hypervitaminosis A may include all of the following: dry and pruritic skin, skin desquamation, erythematous dermatitis, disturbed hair growth, fissures of the lips, pain and tenderness of bones, hyperostosis, headache, papilledema, anorexia, edema, fatigue, irritability, hemorrhage, and neurologic symptoms mimicking those of a brain tumor. *(Hardman et al., p. 1778)*

393. (E) IM administration of 1 mg of vitamin K_1 at birth is required by law in the United States to prevent hypoprothrombinemia of the newborn. *(Hardman et al., p. 1785)*

394. (D) Vitamin D is useful in treating hypocalcemia and secondary hyperparathyroidism caused by chronic renal failure. *(Katzung, pp. 745–746)*

395. (C) Elevated serum 25-hydroxyvitamin D is diagnostic for excess vitamin D. Parathyroid hormone and 1,25-dihydroxyvitamin D production are usually suppressed. Calcium levels are elevated but are not in themselves diagnostic for hypervitaminosis D. *(Hardman et al., pp. 1718–1720)*

396. **(C)** Hydroxylation of the 1 carbon on 25-hydroxyvitamin D_3 is carried out in the kidney, leading to the most active form of the vitamin (calcitriol). Hydroxylation of the 25 carbon is carried out in the liver. *(Katzung, p. 737)*

397. **(B)** PTH decreases calcium excretion by the kidney but increases phosphate excretion, leading to increased serum calcium and decreased serum phosphate levels. Low doses may increase bone formation, whereas high doses increase calcium and phosphate resorption from bone. *(Katzung, p. 738)*

398. **(D)** Calcitriol increases the absorption of both calcium and phosphate from bone and intestine, leading to increased serum levels of both calcium and phosphate. *(Katzung, p. 738)*

399. **(E)** Etidronate causes the development of osteomalacia and increased incidence of fractures when the dosage is raised substantially above 5 mg/kg/d. This same toxicity is not seen with alendronate or pamidronate. *(Katzung, p. 749)*

400. **(A)** Alendronate has been shown to increase bone density and reduce fractures over at least 5 years when used in patients with osteoporosis. *(Katzung, p. 741)*

401. **(E)** The first steps in reducing calcium levels in symptomatic hypercalcemia include rehydration with saline and diuresis with furosemide. Etidronate is useful in treating hypercalcemia of malignancy, whereas calcitonin is often useful as ancillary treatment. Gallium nitrate is approved for management of hypercalcemia of malignancy and acts by inhibiting bone resorption. *(Katzung, pp. 742–743)*

402. **(A)** Oxytocin receptors are coupled to a G-protein (G_q) that activates the calcium–

phosphoinositide-signaling pathway, resulting in increased frequency and force of contraction of uterine smooth muscle. *(Hardman et al., p. 1559)*

403. **(E)** All of the adverse effects listed in this item have been caused by overuse of oxytocin. Hypertensive episodes are due to stimulation of vasopressin receptors by high doses of oxytocin. Water intoxication is due to stimulation of ADH receptors in the kidney. Uterine rupture and damage to the fetus can result from administration of oxytocin to induce labor when the cervix is not completely dilated. *(Katzung, p. 640)*

404. **(C)** To promote fertility in women, GnRH is best administered intravenously by a pump in pulses that promote a physiologic cycle of gonadotropin release. *(Hardman et al., p. 1555)*

405. **(C)** Leuprolide is a synthetic analog of naturally occurring GnRH. When it is administered continuously or in a depot preparation, it has the paradoxic effect of suppressing the release of LH and FSH from the pituitary gland. *(Katzung, p. 942)*

406. **(E)** The symptoms described are most likely the result of ovarian hyperstimulation syndrome (OHSS). This syndrome is believed to be caused by increased ovarian secretion of a substance that increases vascular permeability. *(Hardman et al., p. 1557)*

407. **(A)** In the long term, a depot preparation of leuprolide, which is a long-acting GnRH agonist, inhibits gonadotropin secretion and decreases production of gonadal steroids. In the short term, it may increase gonadotropin secretion. Long-acting GnRH agonists are used for therapy in children with gonadotropin-dependent precocious puberty and as palliative therapy of hormonally responsive tumors such as prostate or breast cancer. *(Hardman et al., p. 1556)*

408. **(D)** T_3 has more thyroid hormone activity than T_4, and reverse T_3 is inactive. *(Katzung, p. 650)*

409. **(A)** The amount of T_4 that is bound by plasma proteins is 99.96%. The amount of T_3 that is bound is 99.6%. *(Katzung, p. 647)*

410. **(E)** Factors that modify the absorption of levothyroxine include food, aluminum-containing antacids, some calcium preparations, sucralfate, iron, and intestinal flora. *(Katzung, p. 646)*

411. **(A)** T_4 is converted within the cell to T_3, which binds to nuclear receptors, resulting in the modulation of the transcription of certain genes. *(Katzung, pp. 648–649)*

412. **(C)** Induction of hepatic enzyme activity by phenytoin, carbamazepine, phenobarbital, rifampin, or rifabutin can result in increased metabolism of both T_3 and T_4 and may require increasing the dose of levothyroxine. *(Katzung, pp. 647–650)*

413. **(A)** Some of the reasons synthetic T_4 is preferred include stability, uniformity of content, ease of laboratory measurement of serum levels, low cost, lack of allergenic foreign protein, and long half-life. *(Katzung, p. 650)*

414. **(E)** Methimazole and propylthiouracil are thioamides used for the treatment of thyrotoxicosis. *(Katzung, p. 651)*

415. **(A)** Methimazole is accumulated by the thyroid gland, and a single 30-mg dose exerts an antithyroid effect for longer than 24 hours. *(Katzung, p. 651)*

416. **(A)** Propylthiouracil inhibits the synthesis of thyroid hormones by blocking iodine organification and to a lesser extent by blocking the coupling of iodotyrosines to form thyroid hormones. It does not block the uptake of iodide by the thyroid gland or the release of thyroid hormones from the gland. *(Katzung, p. 651)*

417. **(D)** Because the thioamides (methimazole and propylthiouracil) block the synthesis but do not block the release of thyroid hormones from the gland, stores of thyroid hormones in

the gland must be depleted before blood levels are affected. The onset of action of the thioamides often occurs after 3 to 4 weeks. *(Katzung, p. 652)*

418. **(B)** Estrogens increase binding of thyroxine by TBG. All of the other pharmacologic agents listed in this item decrease binding. *(Hardman et al., p. 1569)*

419. **(B)** Potassium perchlorate blocks iodide uptake by the thyroid gland by competitive inhibition of the iodide transport mechanism. It is not used often clinically because it has been shown to cause aplastic anemia. *(Katzung, p. 652)*

420. **(D)** The main mechanism of action of pharmacologic doses (> 6 mg per day) of iodides is inhibition of the release of the thyroid hormones, possibly by inhibition of thyroglobulin proteolysis. *(Katzung, p. 652)*

421. **(D)** Glucocorticoid receptors in the cytoplasm are bound to stabilizing proteins. When a glucocorticoid binds to the receptor, an unstable complex results and the stabilizing proteins are released. The glucocorticoid-receptor complex enters the nucleus, where it binds to the glucocorticoid response element on the target gene to regulate transcription. Between 10 and 20% of expressed genes are regulated by glucocorticoids. *(Katzung, pp. 663–664)*

422. **(D)** The effect of glucocorticoids to sensitize cells to the lipolytic effects of the hormones listed in this item is called the permissive effect of glucocorticoids. *(Katzung, p. 664)*

423. **(C)** The responsiveness of vascular and bronchial smooth muscle to the relaxant effects of catecholamines is diminished in the absence and restored in the presence of glucocorticoids. This is called the permissive effect of glucocorticoids. *(Katzung, p. 664)*

424. **(C)** Glucocorticoids increase blood levels of glucose, resulting in the release of insulin from the pancreas, which produces lipogenesis in adipose and other tissues. *(Katzung, p. 665)*

425. **(E)** Supraphysiologic doses of glucocorticoids can cause thinning of the skin, osteoporosis in bone, and muscle weakness due to catabolic effects on these tissues. *(Katzung, p. 665)*

426. **(E)** Circulating neutrophils increase in concentration following a single dose of short-acting glucocorticoid, whereas the other types of leukocytes listed in this item decrease in concentration. *(Katzung, p. 665)*

427. **(E)** All of the functions of macrophages listed in this item are inhibited by glucocorticoids. In addition to macrophages, the ability of lymphocytes to produce interleukin-12 and interferon-gamma, important inducers of T_H1 cell activity and cellular immunity, is inhibited. *(Katzung, p. 665)*

428. **(C)** Glucocorticoids interfere with the effect of vitamin D on calcium absorption from the GI tract. *(Katzung, p. 666)*

429. **(C)** Fludrocortisone is considered a mineralocorticoid, whereas the other steroids listed in this item are glucocorticoids. *(Katzung, p. 666)*

430. **(B)** Dexamethasone is considered a long-acting glucocorticoid. Cortisone, prednisone, and prednisolone are short- to medium-acting glucocorticoids whereas triamcinolone is intermediate acting. *(Katzung, p. 666)*

431. **(A)** Lung maturation in the fetus can be stimulated by betamethasone. This pharmacologic agent is often administered when delivery is anticipated before 34 weeks of gestation. *(Katzung, p. 666)*

432. **(C)** Hydrocortisone has substantial mineralocorticoid activity in contrast to the other corticosteroids listed in this item. *(Katzung, pp. 666, 670)*

433. **(E)** Continuous administration of glucocorticoids tends to cause the face to become

rounded and puffy (moon facies). All of the other conditions listed in this item may accompany iatrogenic Cushing syndrome produced by continuous administration of these agents for longer than 2 weeks. *(Katzung, pp. 669–670)*

434. **(E)** Long-term administration of glucocorticoids, especially in high doses, can lead to all of the complications listed in this item. *(Katzung, p. 670)*

435. **(E)** Estrogen is known to induce the synthesis of progesterone receptors in the uterus. *(Katzung, p. 684)*

436. **(A)** Development of fertility requires FSH and LH, and estrogen interferes with the secretion of these gonadotropins. *(Katzung, pp. 663–664)*

437. **(D)** Estrogen alone significantly increases the risk of endometrial cancer, and addition of a progestin to therapy attenuates this risk. Progestins oppose estrogens' effects on HDL and LDL. *(Katzung, pp. 684–685)*

438. **(E)** Estrogens generally relieve vasomotor symptoms and genital atropy and decrease the risk of osteoporosis in postmenopausal women. Progestins are included in hormone replacement therapy to reduce the risk of endometrial hyperplasia and cancer. *(Katzung, pp. 684–685)*

439. **(E)** The risk of osteoporosis is increased by smoking, being thin, being Caucasian, being inactive, having a low calcium intake, and having a strong family history of osteoporosis. *(Katzung, p. 685)*

440. **(C)** Estrogens have been associated with increased frequency of migraine headaches, breast tenderness, venous thromboembolism, and gallbladder disease, but currently used doses do not increase the risk of hypertension. *(Hardman et al., pp. 1610–1611)*

441. **(C)** Progestins decrease estrogen-driven endometrial proliferation. They also lead to the development of a secretory endometrium and help maintain pregnancy by suppressing menstruation and uterine contractility. The abundant watery secretion of estrogen-stimulated endocervical glands is changed to a scant, viscid product under the influence of progestins. *(Hardman et al., p. 1619)*

442. **(B)** Breakthrough bleeding is the most common adverse effect caused by use of a progestin alone to prevent pregnancy and occurs in up to 25% of patients. *(Katzung, pp. 692–695)*

443. **(A)** The overall incidence of venous thromboembolic disease in women taking oral contraceptives is about three times the risk in women who are not taking these pharmacologic agents. The risk returns to normal within about a month after oral contraceptives are discontinued. A factor contributing to the increased risk may be the decrease in antithrombin III concentrations caused by the contraceptives. *(Katzung, p. 695)*

444. **(B)** If anabolic/androgenic steroids are used too vigorously in children, growth may be rapid at first, but will be arrested before the patient reaches full adult stature because of the effect of the steroids to accelerate epiphyseal closure. *(Katzung, p. 703)*

445. **(D)** Anabolic/androgenic steroids are contraindicated in male patients with carcinoma of the prostate or breast. *(Katzung, pp. 703–704)*

446. **(D)** The principal side effects of the 17α-alkylated androgens are on the liver and include cholestasis, and, rarely, peliosis hepatitis and hepatocellular cancer. *(Hardman et al., p. 1643)*

447. **(A)** As much as 60% of exogenous insulin is cleared by the kidney and 30 to 40% cleared by the liver, presumably by hydrolysis of the disulfide bonds connecting the A and B chains. *(Katzung, pp. 713–714)*

448. **(A)** Insulin inhibits glycogenolysis, the conversion of amino acids to glucose, and the conversion of fatty acids and amino acids to keto acids. It increases the synthesis of

triglycerides and the formation of VLDLs. *(Katzung, p. 715)*

449. **(E)** The durations of action of insulin preparations are classified as follows: Ultra-short-acting, insulin lispro; short-acting, regular; intermediate-acting, Lente and NPH; long-acting, Ultralente. *(Katzung, p. 717)*

450. **(C)** The most common complication of insulin therapy is hypoglycemia. Other complications include insulin allergy, immune insulin resistance, and lipodystrophy at injection sites. *(Katzung, pp. 721–722)*

451. **(D)** The sulfonylureas inhibit potassium efflux through potassium channels in B-cell membranes, causing depolarization of the membranes. The depolarization opens voltage-gated calcium channels, and the resultant calcium influx releases preformed insulin. *(Katzung, pp. 723–724)*

452. **(A)** The thiazolidinediones are selective agonists for the PPARγ, which activates insulin-responsive genes that regulate carbohydrate and lipid metabolism in target tissues. These drugs require insulin to be present for their action. *(Hardman et al., p. 1706)*

453. **(E)** Acarbose and miglitol are competitive inhibitors of intestinal alpha-glucosidases, enzymes that break down starch and disaccharides. The result is that intestinal digestion of these complex carbohydrates is minimized in the upper intestine and deferred to the distal small intestine. The effect on carbohydrate absorption is to lower postmeal excursions in blood glucose concentrations. *(Katzung, pp. 729–730)*

454. **(B)** Repaglinide and nateglinide act on pancreatic beta cells to release insulin. Like sulfonylureas, they close ATP-dependent potassium channels in the cell membranes. *(Hardman et al., pp. 1704–1705)*

455. **(D)** Glyburide, glimepiride, and glipizide are second-generation sulfonylureas. Tolbutamide is a first-generation sulfonylurea. Sec-

ond-generation compounds are generally more potent than first-generation agents and should be used with caution in patients in whom hypoglycemia would be especially dangerous, such as patients with cardiovascular disease and the elderly. *(Katzung, pp. 725–727)*

456. **(E)** Rosiglitazone and pioglitazone are thiazolidinediones. An earlier member of this group, troglitazone, was withdrawn because of severe liver toxicity, resulting in a number of deaths. Rosiglitazone and pioglitazone do not appear to have the same toxic potential. *(Katzung, pp. 728–729)*

457. **(C)** The most frequent adverse effect of glyburide is hypoglycemia. It produces few other adverse effects. *(Katzung, p. 726)*

458. **(E)** Repaglinide is a member of the meglitinide group, and its rapid onset of action and short duration make it suitable for administration just before meals to control post-

meal blood glucose excursions. *(Katzung, p. 727)*

459. **(B)** The most common adverse reactions to alpha-glucosidase inhibitors are GI disturbances due to undigested carbohydrates reaching the colon and then being fermented into short-chain fatty acids, resulting in the release of gas. These disturbances include flatulence, diarrhea, and abdominal pain. *(Katzung, p. 730)*

460. **(A)** Metabolism of carbohydrate consumes thiamine. Therefore, thiamine should be administered before or along with dextrose-containing fluids to any patient whose nutritional status may be marginal. *(Hardman et al., p. 1755)*

461. **(C)** Nicotinic acid and nicotinamide and their derivatives can be used for prevention and therapy of pellagra, the clinical condition caused by nicotinic acid deficiency. *(Hardman et al., pp. 1758–1759)*

CHAPTER 6

Chemotherapeutic Agents
Questions

DIRECTIONS (Questions 462 through 563): Each of the numbered items or incomplete statements in this section is followed by answers or by completions of the statement. Select the ONE lettered answer or completion that is BEST in each case.

462. Which of the following beta-lactam antibiotics is most resistant to staphylococcal beta-lactamases?

(A) amoxicillin
(B) ampicillin
(C) oxacillin
(D) penicillin G
(E) ticarcillin

463. Which of the following features best represents an advantage of ampicillin over penicillin G?

(A) improved activity against gram-negative cocci
(B) improved activity against gram-negative rods
(C) improved activity against gram-positive organisms
(D) improved activity against non–beta-lactamase-producing anaerobes
(E) improved resistance against beta-lactamases

464. Beta-lactam antibiotics are bactericidal due to their interference with which of the following processes?

(A) N-acetylation of glucosamine
(B) N-acetylation of muramic acid
(C) polymerization of monosaccharides

(D) ribosomal protein biosynthesis
(E) transpeptidation reaction

465. Which of the following mechanisms is LEAST likely to contribute to bacterial resistance to penicillins and other beta-lactams?

(A) impaired penetration of the antibiotic through the outer membrane
(B) inactivation of the antibiotic by beta-lactamase
(C) induction of transpeptidase
(D) modification of target penicillin-binding proteins
(E) the presence of an efflux pump

466. Which of the following penicillins is the most nephrotoxic?

(A) amoxicillin
(B) ampicillin
(C) cloxacillin
(D) dicloxacillin
(E) methicillin

467. Which of the following penicillins is cleared primarily by the kidneys and therefore must be administered in a lower dose in patients with compromised renal function?

(A) amoxicillin
(B) cloxacillin
(C) dicloxacillin
(D) nafcillin
(E) oxacillin

468. Clavulanic acid belongs to which of the following groups of drugs?

(A) beta-lactam antibiotics

(B) beta-lactamase inhibitors

(C) cytochrome P450 inducers

(D) cytochrome P450 inhibitors

(E) inhibitors of renal tubular secretion of weak acids

469. Which of the following statements about penicillins is (are) true?

(A) All penicillins are cross-reacting and cross-sensitizing.

(B) Most of the serious adverse reactions to penicillins are caused by hypersensitivity.

(C) The antigenic determinates that are most responsible for hypersensitivity reactions to penicillins are degradation products.

(D) all of the above

(E) none of the above

470. Of the patients who have previously been given penicillin without incident, what percentage will have an allergic reaction when given penicillin?

(A) fewer than 1%

(B) 1 to 5%

(C) 5 to 10%

(D) 10 to 15%

(E) 15 to 20%

471. Which of the following antibiotics is most susceptible to hydrolysis by beta-lactamases?

(A) axetil

(B) cefaclor

(C) cefprozil

(D) cefuroxime

(E) loracarbef

472. Which of the following third-generation cephalosporins achieves concentrations in the cerebrospinal fluid (CSF) sufficient to inhibit most pathogens except, perhaps, *Pseudomonas*?

(A) cefixime

(B) cefoperazone

(C) cefpodoxime proxetil

(D) ceftibuten

(E) ceftriaxone

473. Which of the following antibiotics is excreted mainly through the biliary tract and therefore does not need any dosage adjustment for renal insufficiency?

(A) cefazolin

(B) cefotaxime

(C) cefoxitin

(D) ceftazidime

(E) ceftriaxone

474. Beta-lactamase inhibitors are most effective against beta-lactamases produced by which of the following bacteria?

(A) *Citrobacter*

(B) *Enterobacter*

(C) *Pseudomonas*

(D) *Serratia*

(E) *Staphylococcus*

475. The antibiotic action of erythromycin is due to its interference with which of the following processes?

(A) gene transcription

(B) N-acetylation of glucosamine

(C) N-acetylation of muramic acid

(D) polymerization of monosaccharides

(E) ribosomal protein biosynthesis

476. What is the reason tetracyclines do not inhibit protein biosynthesis in mammalian cells?

(A) An active efflux mechanism in mammalian cells prevents intracellular accumulation of the drug.

(B) Mammalian genes code for proteins that are different from bacterial proteins.

(C) Tetracyclines do not bind to mammalian ribosomes.

(D) Tetracyclines do not block binding of amino acid–charged transfer RNA (tRNA) to the acceptor site of the ribosome–messenger RNA (mRNA) complex in mammalian cells.

(E) Tetracyclines do not penetrate across mammalian cell membranes.

477. Which of the following mechanisms has (have) been described for causing bacterial resistance to tetracyclines?

(A) enzymatic inactivation of the drug
(B) impaired influx of the drug or increased efflux by an active transport system
(C) interference with binding of the drug to the bacterial ribosome
(D) all of the above
(E) none of the above

478. Which of the following factors is (are) known to interfere with absorption of tetracyclines from the intestine?

(A) alkaline pH
(B) antacids
(C) dairy products
(D) divalent cations
(E) all of the above

479. What is the most likely effect of carbamazepine, phenytoin, barbiturates, and chronic alcohol ingestion on the pharmacokinetics of doxycycline?

(A) They increase free levels in the plasma by displacement of doxycycline from plasma proteins.
(B) They prolong the half-life by inhibition of hepatic enzymes.
(C) They prolong the half-life by interference with the excretion of doxycycline by the kidney.
(D) They reduce plasma levels by interference with absorption from the intestine.
(E) They shorten the half-life by induction of hepatic enzymes.

480. Which of the following tetracyclines is most suitable for administration to patients with renal insufficiency?

(A) chlortetracycline
(B) demeclocycline

(C) doxycycline
(D) methacycline
(E) oxytetracycline

481. Which of the following tetracyclines has the longest duration of action?

(A) chlortetracycline
(B) demeclocycline
(C) minocycline
(D) oxytetracycline
(E) tetracycline

482. When a tetracycline is given during pregnancy, which tissue will most likely be affected adversely in the fetus?

(A) bone
(B) heart
(C) kidney
(D) liver
(E) skeletal muscle

483. Which of the following statements best describes the interaction of erythromycin or its metabolites with warfarin?

(A) Erythromycin metabolites directly inhibit the biosynthesis of vitamin K–dependent clotting factors, leading to an enhancement of the anticoagulant effects of warfarin.
(B) Erythromycin metabolites lower plasma levels of warfarin by inducing hepatic enzymes that metabolize the anticoagulant.
(C) Erythromycin metabolites raise plasma levels of warfarin by inhibiting hepatic enzymes that metabolize the anticoagulant.
(D) Erythromycin raises plasma levels of unbound warfarin by displacing the anticoagulant from plasma proteins.
(E) Erythromycin raises plasma levels of warfarin by increasing the bioavailability of the anticoagulant.

484. How is the pharmacology of clarithromycin different from erythromycin?

(A) Clarithromycin has better acid stability and oral absorption.

(B) Clarithromycin has fewer drug interactions.

(C) Erythromycin-resistant staphylococci are susceptible to clarithromycin.

(D) Erythromycin-resistant streptococci are susceptible to clarithromycin.

(E) all of the above

485. Cross-resistance is complete between linezolid and which of the following antibiotics?

(A) clindamycin

(B) erythromycin

(C) quinupristin–dalfopristin

(D) all of the above

(E) none of the above

486. The antibiotic activity of type B streptogramins is due to blockade of which of the following processes?

(A) gene transcription

(B) N-acetylation of glucosamine

(C) N-acetylation of muramic acid

(D) polymerization of monosaccharides

(E) ribosomal protein biosynthesis

487. Which of the following antibiotics has the greatest liability for producing toxic effects on the bone marrow?

(A) chloramphenicol

(B) clindamycin

(C) erythromycin

(D) streptogramins

(E) tetracyclines

488. Aminoglycoside antibiotics are useful mainly against which type(s) of microorganisms?

(A) aerobic gram-negative microorganisms

(B) aerobic gram-positive microorganisms

(C) anaerobic gram-negative microorganisms

(D) anaerobic gram-positive microorganisms

(E) both aerobic and anaerobic gram-positive microorganisms

489. Which of the following accurately describe(s) the effect(s) of streptomycin on bacterial ribosomal protein biosynthesis?

(A) It causes misreading of mRNA.

(B) It causes polysomes to break up into nonfunctional monosomes.

(C) It interferes with the initiation complex of peptide formation.

(D) all of the above

(E) none of the above

490. Which of the following best describes the principal type of resistance to aminoglycosides encountered clinically?

(A) adenylylation, acetylation, or phosphorylation of the aminoglycoside catalyzed by a transferase enzyme or enzymes, resulting in inactivation of the antibiotic

(B) deletion or alteration of the receptor protein on the 30S ribosomal subunit

(C) efflux of the aminoglycoside due to an active pump

(D) impairment of the entry of the aminoglycoside into the cell

(E) induction of new proteins that competitively inhibit aminoglycoside binding to the 30S ribosomal subunit

491. Which of the following statements most accurately applies to aminoglycosides?

(A) After intravenous (IV) administration, they are rapidly distributed to most tissues in concentrations ranging from 60 to 90% of plasma levels.

(B) In order to achieve high levels in CSF, they must be administered by intrathecal or intraventricular injection.

(C) It is not necessary to adjust the dosage for patients with renal impairment.

(D) They are rapidly metabolized to inactive products by hepatic enzymes.

(E) They are well absorbed from the gastrointestinal (GI) tract.

492. Which of the following factors is (are) known to increase the likelihood of aminoglycoside-induced nephrotoxicity?

(A) The patient has renal insufficiency.
(B) The patient is elderly.
(C) The patient is receiving concurrent treatment with furosemide.
(D) The patient is receiving concurrent treatment with vancomycin.
(E) all of the above

493. Which of the following adverse reactions is most likely to occur in response to aminoglycosides?

(A) liver toxicity
(B) ototoxicity
(C) Parkinson's disease–like syndrome
(D) venous thrombosis
(E) visual disturbances

494. High doses of aminoglycosides are most likely to produce which of the following adverse effects?

(A) cardiac arrhythmias
(B) central nervous system (CNS) depression
(C) elevated blood pressure
(D) neuromuscular blockade
(E) stroke

495. What is the most serious toxic effect of streptomycin?

(A) cardiac arrhythmias
(B) CNS depression
(C) cholestatic jaundice
(D) ocular disturbances
(E) vestibular dysfunction

496. Gentamicin belongs to which class of antibiotics?

(A) aminoglycosides
(B) beta-lactam antibiotics
(C) macrolides
(D) quinolones
(E) streptogramins

497. Which of the following mechanisms is (are) known to be part of the reason combination of gentamicin with penicillin or vancomycin produces a potent bactericidal effect against streptococci and enterococci?

(A) The binding site on the 50S ribosomal subunit has enhanced affinity for gentamicin.
(B) The efflux of gentamicin by an active pump is reduced.
(C) The transferase enzyme or enzymes that inactivate gentamicin are inhibited.
(D) The uptake of gentamicin into the cell is enhanced.
(E) all of the above

498. Which of the following antibiotics is least absorbed from the GI tract upon oral administration?

(A) amoxicillin
(B) ampicillin
(C) clarithromycin
(D) doxycycline
(E) neomycin

499. Which of the following antibiotics is most similar to gentamicin in pharmacokinetic properties and antibacterial spectrum?

(A) azithromycin
(B) clarithromycin
(C) moxifloxacin
(D) tobramycin
(E) vancomycin

500. Once-daily aminoglycoside dosing is often preferred over multiple daily dosing for which of the following reasons?

(A) Aminoglycosides have a significant postantibiotic effect against bacteria.
(B) Aminoglycosides have concentration-dependent killing rather than time-dependent killing.
(C) Toxicity tends to depend on the time that the aminoglycoside concentration is above a certain threshold.
(D) all of the above
(E) none of the above

501. The chemical structure of sulfonamides is most similar to which of the following compounds?

    (A) para-aminobenzoic acid (PABA)
    (B) pantothenic acid
    (C) tetrahydrofolic acid
    (D) gamma-aminobutyric acid (GABA)
    (E) gamma-carboxyglutamic acid

502. Which of the following statements best describes the antimicrobial activity of sulfonamides?

    (A) They are bactericidal for both gram-positive and gram-negative bacteria.
    (B) They are bactericidal for gram-negative bacteria only.
    (C) They are bactericidal for gram-positive bacteria only.
    (D) They are bacteriostatic for both gram-positive and gram-negative bacteria.
    (E) They are bacteriostatic for gram-positive bacteria only.

503. Which of the following statements accurately reflect(s) the mechanism(s) by which bacteria become resistant to sulfonamides?

    (A) Mutations cause a loss of permeability of the cell membrane to sulfonamides.
    (B) Mutations cause formation of a folic acid–synthesizing enzyme that has a low affinity for sulfonamides.
    (C) Mutations cause overproduction of PABA.
    (D) all of the above
    (E) none of the above

504. Which of the following sulfonamides has the longest duration of action?

    (A) sulfacytine
    (B) sulfadiazine
    (C) sulfadoxine
    (D) sulfamethizole
    (E) sulfamethoxazole

505. Which drug or drug combination is administered by the intravenous route most often?

    (A) sulfadoxine
    (B) sulfamethoxazole
    (C) sulfisoxazole
    (D) trimethoprim–sulfadoxine
    (E) trimethoprim–sulfamethoxazole

506. Which of the following statements LEAST accurately reflects the properties of sulfadiazine?

    (A) It crosses the placenta and is distributed to the fetus.
    (B) It is absorbed from the stomach and small intestine after oral administration.
    (C) It is not distributed in therapeutic levels to the CSF.
    (D) It is readily distributed to the lungs.
    (E) When combined with pyrimethamine, the combination has synergistic action against toxoplasmosis.

507. Which of the following statements most accurately describes a property of sulfadoxine?

    (A) It appears in the plasma mainly as free drug because there is very little binding to plasma proteins.
    (B) It is a relatively short-acting sulfonamide.
    (C) It is not well absorbed from the intestine after oral administration.
    (D) It is rapidly excreted by the kidney.
    (E) The free drug undergoes extensive tubular reabsorption in the kidney.

508. Which of the following statements LEAST accurately reflects the properties of sulfasalazine?

    (A) It has a therapeutic effect similar to olsalazine, although it may not be as well tolerated.
    (B) It is split by intestinal microflora to yield 5-aminosalicylate, which produces a beneficial anti-inflammatory effect.

(C) It is split by intestinal microflora, yielding sulfapyridine as one of its products.

(D) It is useful in treating inflammatory bowel disease.

(E) It is well absorbed from the intestine after oral administration.

509. Which of the following pharmacologic agents is (are) cross-allergenic with sulfonamides?

(A) carbonic anhydrase inhibitors

(B) furosemide

(C) sulfonylurea hypoglycemic agents

(D) thiazide diuretics

(E) all of the above

510. In addition to the administration of fluids, what agent(s) is (are) useful in treating nephrotoxicity caused by sulfadiazine?

(A) folinic acid

(B) probenecid

(C) sodium bicarbonate

(D) sulfinpyrazone

(E) all of the above

511. Where in the body is trimethoprim concentrated when therapeutic doses are given?

(A) adipose tissue

(B) CSF

(C) inner ear

(D) liver

(E) prostatic fluid and vaginal fluid

512. Which of the following toxic reactions would most likely be produced by trimethoprim?

(A) cholestatic jaundice

(B) crystalluria

(C) megaloblastic anemia

(D) tinnitus

(E) venous thrombosis

513. Which of the following alterations is (are) known to occur resulting in resistance to trimethoprim?

(A) decreased bacterial cell permeability

(B) overproduction of bacterial dihydrofolate reductase

(C) production of a modified dihydrofolate reductase with a lower affinity for the drug

(D) all of the above

(E) none of the above

514. To what group of drugs does ciprofloxacin belong?

(A) aminoglycosides

(B) beta-lactam antibiotics

(C) fluoroquinolones

(D) macrolides

(E) sulfonamides

515. Important quinolones are synthetic fluorinated analogs of what compound?

(A) nalidixic acid

(B) PABA

(C) pantothenic acid

(D) tetrahydrofolic acid

(E) GABA

516. The antimicrobial activity of ciprofloxacin is caused by its inhibition of which of the following bacterial enzymes?

(A) dihydrofolate reductase

(B) dihydropteroate synthase

(C) enolpyruvate transferase

(D) RNA polymerase

(E) topoisomerase II and topoisomerase IV

517. Of the following antibiotics, which one is the most active against gram-negative bacteria?

(A) ciprofloxacin

(B) enoxacin

(C) levofloxacin

(D) lomefloxacin

(E) ofloxacin

518. Which of the following is (are) the most common adverse effect(s) caused by fluoroquinolones?

    (A) CNS depression
    (B) cholestatic jaundice
    (C) nausea, vomiting, and diarrhea
    (D) nephrotoxicity
    (E) skin rashes

519. Which of the following drugs has the greatest potential for adverse drug interaction if administered concomitantly with fluoroquinolones?

    (A) carbamazepine
    (B) insulin
    (C) metformin
    (D) theophylline
    (E) warfarin

520. Four of the drugs listed below are first-line agents for treatment of tuberculosis and one is a second-line agent. Which one is the second-line agent?

    (A) ciprofloxacin
    (B) ethambutol
    (C) isoniazid
    (D) pyrazinamide
    (E) rifampin

521. Which of the following agents can reverse the peripheral neuropathy caused by isoniazid?

    (A) ascorbic acid
    (B) folate
    (C) niacin
    (D) pyridoxine
    (E) thiamine

522. Which of the following is the main cause of resistance of mycobacteria to rifampin?

    (A) decreased penetration of rifampin into the bacterial cell
    (B) increased efflux of rifampin from the bacterial cell by an active pump
    (C) increased formation of an enzyme that inactivates rifampin

    (D) mutation preventing the binding of rifampin to RNA polymerase
    (E) mutation resulting in overexpression of RNA polymerase

523. Which of the following is the most common serious adverse event associated with use of ethambutol?

    (A) bone marrow suppression
    (B) hepatitis
    (C) nephritis
    (D) psychotic reaction
    (E) visual disturbance

524. Which of the following antimycobacterial drugs exerts its antimicrobial activity mainly against intracellular organisms that have been taken up by macrophages?

    (A) ethambutol
    (B) isoniazid
    (C) pyrazinamide
    (D) rifampin
    (E) streptomycin

525. Which of the following drugs exerts its antimycobacterial activity by interfering with the synthesis of mycolic acids, which are essential components of mycobacterial cell walls?

    (A) ethambutol
    (B) isoniazid
    (C) pyrazinamide
    (D) rifampin
    (E) streptomycin

526. Which of the following drugs exerts its antimycobacterial activity by interfering with the synthesis of arabinoglycan, which is an essential component of mycobacterial cell walls?

    (A) ethambutol
    (B) isoniazid
    (C) pyrazinamide
    (D) rifampin
    (E) streptomycin

527. Which of the following toxicities represents the most serious toxic reaction to amphotericin B?

    (A) hematologic toxicity
    (B) liver toxicity
    (C) neuropathy
    (D) ototoxicity
    (E) renal toxicity

528. Which of the following mechanisms accounts for the antifungal activity of amphotericin B?

    (A) formation of pores in the cell membrane
    (B) inhibition of cytochrome P450 enzymes
    (C) inhibition of DNA and RNA synthesis
    (D) inhibition of ribosomal protein biosynthesis
    (E) inhibition of squalene epoxidase

529. Which of the following mechanisms accounts for the antifungal activity of flucytosine?

    (A) formation of pores in the cell membrane
    (B) inhibition of cytochrome P450 enzymes
    (C) inhibition of DNA and RNA synthesis
    (D) inhibition of ribosomal protein biosynthesis
    (E) inhibition of squalene epoxidase

530. Which of the following mechanisms accounts for the antifungal activity of terbinafine?

    (A) formation of pores in the cell membrane
    (B) inhibition of cytochrome P450 enzymes
    (C) inhibition of DNA and RNA synthesis
    (D) inhibition of ribosomal protein biosynthesis
    (E) inhibition of squalene epoxidase

531. Which of the following drugs is poorly absorbed from the intestine and has the least systemic antifungal activity when administered by the oral route?

    (A) amphotericin B
    (B) flucytosine
    (C) itraconazole
    (D) ketoconazole
    (E) terbinafine

532. Which of the following drugs is available in lipid delivery vehicles to permit the use of effective doses of the drug, but with reduced toxicity to the patient?

    (A) amphotericin B
    (B) flucytosine
    (C) itraconazole
    (D) ketoconazole
    (E) terbinafine

533. Which of the following steps in viral replication is (are) targeted by acyclovir?

    (A) DNA synthesis
    (B) packaging and assembly of the viron
    (C) protein synthesis by host polysome
    (D) uncoating of the viral DNA
    (E) all of the above

534. Which of the following represent(s) mechanism(s) by which resistance to acyclovir develops?

    (A) alteration of neuraminidase
    (B) alteration of proteases
    (C) alteration of reverse transcriptase
    (D) alteration of thymidine kinase
    (E) all of the above

535. An HIV-infected patient is receiving ganciclovir for treatment of cytomegalovirus retinitis. What is the most likely type of drug interaction that may occur if zidovudine is used concomitantly.

    (A) accumulation of zidovudine due to cytochrome P450 inhibition by ganciclovir
    (B) accumulation of zidovudine due to decreased biliary excretion caused by ganciclovir
    (C) additive CNS toxicity
    (D) additive myelosuppression
    (E) lower systemic levels of zidovudine due to cytochrome P450 induction by ganciclovir

536. Which of the following toxic reactions represents the primary adverse effect of intravenous cidofovir?

    (A) CNS symptoms
    (B) hepatotoxicity
    (C) nephrotoxicity
    (D) ototoxicity
    (E) skin rash

537. Which of the following represents the primary mechanism targeted by fomivirsen by which the drug inhibits virus replication?

    (A) inhibition of DNA synthesis
    (B) inhibition of packaging and assembly of the viron
    (C) inhibition of protein synthesis
    (D) inhibition of uncoating of the virion
    (E) inhibition of viral release from the host cell

538. To which of the following groups of drugs does zidovudine belong?

    (A) antiherpes and anticytomegalovirus agents
    (B) nonnucleoside reverse transcriptase inhibitors
    (C) nucleoside reverse transcriptase inhibitors
    (D) nucleotide reverse transcriptase inhibitors
    (E) protease inhibitors

539. Which of the following represents the major clinical toxicity associated with didanosine therapy?

    (A) cardiomyopathy
    (B) hepatotoxicity
    (C) myelosuppression
    (D) nephrotoxicity
    (E) pancreatitis

540. Which of the following represents the major clinical toxicity associated with zalcitabine therapy?

    (A) hepatotoxicity
    (B) myelosuppression

    (C) nephrotoxicity
    (D) pancreatitis
    (E) peripheral neuropathy

541. Which of the following represents the most important limitation to the ease of administration of ritonavir?

    (A) effect of food on absorption from the GI tract
    (B) interactions with other drugs
    (C) nephrotoxicity
    (D) pancreatitis
    (E) poor bioavailability ($< 20\%$)

542. Which of the following protease inhibitors has the highest penetration into the CSF?

    (A) amprenavir
    (B) indinavir
    (C) nelfinavir
    (D) ritonavir
    (E) saquinavir

543. What is the primary mechanism by which amantadine and rimantadine inhibit the replication of influenza A virus?

    (A) inhibition of DNA synthesis
    (B) inhibition of packaging and assembly of the virion
    (C) inhibition of protein synthesis
    (D) inhibition of reverse transcriptase
    (E) inhibition of uncoating of the viral RNA

544. What is the primary mechanism by which didanosine inhibits viral replication?

    (A) inhibition of RNA synthesis
    (B) inhibition of packaging and assembly of the virion
    (C) inhibition of protein synthesis
    (D) inhibition of reverse transcriptase
    (E) inhibition of uncoating of the viral RNA

545. Which of the following is the main reason for giving ritonavir along with saquinavir?

    (A) to decrease the development of resistance
    (B) to decrease the toxicity of the saquinavir

(C) to increase the concentrations of saquinavir reaching the systemic circulation

(D) to inhibit viral replication by two different mechanisms of action

(E) to reduce GI symptoms associated with saquinavir

546. Which of the following drugs is most effective against extraintestinal infections by *Entamoeba histolytica*?

(A) diloxanide furoate
(B) iodoquinol
(C) mefloquine
(D) metronidazole
(E) paromomycin sulfate

547. Which of the following drugs or drug combinations is most effective therapy for *Pneumocystis carinii* pneumonia?

(A) furazolidone
(B) metronidazole
(C) paromomycin
(D) tetracycline
(E) trimethoprim plus sulfamethoxazole

548. Which of the following represents the greatest limitation in the usefulness of chloroquine for the treatment of *Plasmodium falciparum* infection?

(A) hepatotoxicity
(B) nephrotoxicity
(C) poor absorption of the phosphate salt from the GI tract
(D) poor distribution of the drug to the tissues
(E) resistant strains

549. Which of the following is the drug of choice for eradication of dormant hepatic stages of *Plasmodium vivax* and *Plasmodium ovale*?

(A) amodiaquine
(B) chloroquine
(C) mefloquine
(D) primaquine
(E) quinine

550. Which of the following antimalarial drugs act by inhibition of plasmodial dihydrofolate reductase?

(A) amodiaquine
(B) artemisinin
(C) mefloquine
(D) pyrimethamine
(E) quinine

551. Which of the following drugs should be avoided during therapy with metronidazole?

(A) alcohol
(B) diloxanide furoate
(C) iodoquinol
(D) paromomycin
(E) all of the above

552. Which of the following classes of anticancer drugs is cell cycle nonspecific?

(A) alkylating agents
(B) antimetabolites
(C) bleomycin peptide antibiotics
(D) plant alkaloids
(E) podophyllin alkaloids

553. P-glycoprotein is a

(A) cellular glycoprotein that transports foreign molecules
(B) component of the cell membrane that is primarily structural in function
(C) component of the endoplasmic reticulum that facilitates drug biotransformation
(D) glycoprotein involved primarily in cell signaling mechanisms
(E) glycoprotein that binds to and inhibits certain transcription factors

554. Which of the following toxic reactions represents the major toxicity produced by alkylating agents used for therapy of cancer?

(A) hepatotoxicity
(B) nephrotoxicity
(C) peripheral neuropathy
(D) reduction of erythrocyte count
(E) reduction of white blood cell count

555. In which of the following stages of breast cancer is chemotherapy as adjuvant to surgery (e.g., with cyclophosphamide–methotrexate–fluorouracil or fluorouracil-doxorubicin–cyclophosphamide) of most benefit?

(A) Stage I
(B) Stage II with one to three involved lymph nodes
(C) Stage II with four or more involved lymph nodes
(D) Stage III
(E) Stage IV

556. Approximately what percentage of patients with nonseminomatous testicular neoplasms enter complete remission in response to combination chemotherapy with cisplatin, vinblastine, and bleomycin?

(A) 0%
(B) 10%
(C) 30%
(D) 50%
(E) 90%

557. Which of the following classes of anticancer drugs is cell cycle specific?

(A) alkylating agents
(B) antibiotics
(C) cisplatin
(D) nitrosoureas
(E) plant alkaloids

558. For which of the following anticancer agents does intracellular formation of polyglutamate derivatives appear to be important?

(A) cytarabine
(B) fluorouracil
(C) mercaptopurine
(D) methotrexate
(E) vinblastine

559. Which of the following anticancer drugs causes cell death mainly by alkylations of DNA in the nucleus as well as alkylations of sulfhydryl, amino, hydroxyl, carboxyl, and phosphate groups of other cellular nucleophiles?

(A) chlorambucil
(B) cytarabine
(C) doxorubicin
(D) methotrexate
(E) vincristine

560. Which of the following anticancer drugs is converted in the body to a metabolite that blocks DNA synthesis by competitive inhibition of DNA polymerase?

(A) cytarabine
(B) etoposide
(C) melphalan
(D) paclitaxel
(E) tamoxifen

561. Which of the following anticancer drugs interrupts the mitotic cycle mainly by causing arrest in metaphase?

(A) cisplatin
(B) daunorubicin
(C) fluorouracil
(D) gemcitabine
(E) vinblastine

562. Which of the following anticancer drugs block progression through the cell cycle mainly by inhibition of topoisomerase II?

(A) chlorambucil
(B) dactinomycin
(C) etoposide
(D) methotrexate
(E) procarbazine

563. Which of the following anticancer drugs inhibits DNA-dependent RNA synthesis mainly as a result of its intercalation between adjacent guanine–cytosine base pairs in double-stranded DNA?

(A) dactinomycin
(B) flutamide
(C) methotrexate
(D) paclitaxel
(E) vinblastine

Answers and Explanations

462. (C) The penicillins that are resistant to staphylococcal beta-lactamase include methicillin, nafcillin, and isoxazolyl penicillins such as oxacillin, cloxacillin, and dicloxacillin. *(Katzung, pp. 754–761)*

463. (B) Penicillin G is effective against gram-positive organisms, gram-negative cocci, and non–beta-lactamase-producing anaerobes. However, it has little activity against gram-negative rods. Ampicillin has greater activity against gram-negative organisms than penicillin G. *(Katzung, pp. 754–755)*

464. (E) Beta-lactam antibiotics interfere with bacterial cell wall synthesis by blocking the transpeptidation reaction in peptidoglycan synthesis. *(Katzung, p. 755)*

465. (C) There are four general mechanisms of resistance to beta-lactam antibiotics, and these are listed in this item. Induction of transpeptidase does not appear to be a mechanism by which resistance is conferred. *(Katzung, pp. 755–757)*

466. (E) Use of methicillin has been discontinued because of its nephrotoxicity. *(Katzung, pp. 757–760)*

467. (A) The dosage of amoxicillin must be reduced when creatinine clearance falls to 10 mLr/min. Nafcillin is cleared primarily by biliary excretion and oxacillin, dicloxacillin, and cloxacillin are cleared by both the kidney and biliary excretion, and therefore the dosages do not need to be adjusted for renal function. *(Katzung, pp. 758–760)*

468. (B) Clavulanic acid, sulbactam, and tazobactam are beta-lactamase inhibitors. They are included in combination with ampicillin, amoxicillin, ticarcillin, and piperacillin to extend the activity of these penicillins to include some beta-lactamase–producing strains of bacteria. *(Katzung, p. 761)*

469. (D) It is true that hypersensitivity reactions account for most of the adverse reactions to penicillins, that all penicillins are cross-reacting and cross-sensitizing, and that degradation products are the main antigenic determinants. *(Katzung, p. 761)*

470. (A) Of the patients who have received penicillin previously without incident, fewer than 1% will have allergic reactions to penicillin. *(Katzung, p. 761)*

471. (B) All of the antibiotics listed in this item are orally effective second-generation cephalosporins. Cefaclor is more susceptible to hydrolysis by beta-lactamases than the other agents in this group. *(Katzung, p. 764)*

472. (E) Except for cefoperazone, cefixime, ceftibuten, and cefpodoxime proxetil, the third-generation cephalosporins penetrate body fluids and tissues well, including the CSF. *(Katzung, pp. 764–765)*

473. (E) Most cephalosporins are excreted through the kidney and need to be dosage adjusted for renal insufficiency. Ceftriaxone and cefoperazone are exceptions to this rule. *(Katzung, pp. 765–766)*

474. **(E)** Beta-lactamase inhibitors are most active against Ambler class A beta-lactamases. Organisms producing this type of beta-lactamase include staphylococci, *Haemophilus influenzae*, *Neisseria gonorrhoeae*, *Salmonella*, *Shigella*, *Escherichia coli*, and *Klebsiella pneumoniae*. These inhibitors are not very effective against class C beta-lactamases produced by *Enterobacter*, *Citrobacter*, *Serratia*, and *Pseudomonas*. *(Katzung, p. 767)*

475. **(E)** Macrolides interfere with protein biosynthesis by preventing translocation of peptidyl tRNA from the acceptor site to the donor site on the bacterial ribosome. *(Katzung, p. 775)*

476. **(A)** In mammalian cells, there is an active efflux mechanism that prevents intracellular accumulation of tetracycline antibiotics. *(Katzung, p. 775)*

477. **(D)** All three mechanism listed have been described by which bacterial resistance to tetracyclines is produced. The most important of these is efflux of the drug by an active pump. *(Katzung, p. 777)*

478. **(E)** All of the factors listed in this item are known to impair the absorption of tetracyclines. In addition, food can decrease absorption of all the tetracyclines except doxycycline and minocycline. *(Katzung, p. 777)*

479. **(E)** The drugs listed in this item can shorten the half-life of doxycycline 50% by induction of hepatic enzymes. *(Katzung, p. 777)*

480. **(C)** In contrast with other tetracyclines, doxycycline is eliminated by nonrenal mechanisms and therefore requires no dosage adjustment in patients with renal insufficiency. *(Katzung, p. 777)*

481. **(C)** The classification of tetracyclines based on their half-lives is as follows: Short-acting (6 to 8 hours)—chlortetracycline, tetracycline, and oxytetracycline; intermediate-acting (12 hours)—demeclocycline and methacycline; and long-acting (16 to 18 hours)—doxycycline and minocycline. *(Katzung, p. 777)*

482. **(A)** Tetracyclines bind readily to calcium deposited in newly formed bone. When given during pregnancy, it can cause deformity of bone or growth inhibition in the fetus. It also can be deposited in fetal teeth, causing fluorescence, discoloration, and enamel dysplasia. *(Katzung, p. 778)*

483. **(C)** Erythromycin metabolites can inhibit hepatic cytochrome P450 enzymes, causing an increase in plasma concentrations of warfarin and other drugs, including theophylline, cyclosporine, and methylprednisolone. *(Katzung, p. 780)*

484. **(A)** Clarithromycin is a semisynthetic derivative of erythromycin that has better acid stability and oral absorption compared to erythromycin. *(Katzung, p. 780)*

485. **(E)** Linezolid acts by preventing formation of the ribosome complex that initiates protein synthesis. It is not cross-resistant with other drug classes because of its unique binding site located on the 23S ribosomal RNA of the 50S subunit. *(Katzung, p. 782)*

486. **(E)** Quinupristin is a type B streptogramin. These agents block ribosomal protein synthesis by preventing translocation of peptidyl tRNA from the acceptor site to the donor site on the 50S ribosomal subunit. The combination of quinupristin with dalfopristin (type A streptogramin) is bactericidal for most bacteria. *(Katzung, pp. 776, 782)*

487. **(A)** Chloramphenicol affects bone marrow in two ways. It can cause a dose-related toxicity that results in anemia, leukopenia, or thrombocytopenia. It can also cause aplastic anemia, which is an idiosyncratic reaction unrelated to dose. The latter effect is rare, but it can be fatal. *(Katzung, p. 776)*

488. **(A)** Aminoglycosides are bactericidal antibiotics that are useful mainly against aerobic gram-negative organisms. *(Katzung, p. 784)*

489. **(D)** Streptomycin binds to S12 ribosomal proteins on the 30S subunit and inhibits pro-

tein biosynthesis in at least the three ways described in this item. *(Katzung, p. 784)*

490. **(A)** Inactivation of the aminoglycoside is the principal mechanism of resistance encountered clinically. Other mechanisms that have been described include impaired entry of the aminoglycoside into the cell and deletion or alteration of the receptor protein on the 30S ribosomal subunit. *(Katzung, pp. 784–785)*

491. **(B)** Aminoglycosides are highly polar compounds that are not well absorbed from the intestine and are not well distributed to most tissues even after IV administration. Since they are cleared mainly by the kidney, the dose must be adjusted when renal function is impaired. *(Katzung, p. 785)*

492. **(E)** Nephrotoxicity caused by aminoglycosides is more prevalent in patients who are elderly, experiencing renal insufficiency, receiving loop diuretics, or receiving other nephrotoxic antibiotics such as vancomycin or amphotericin. *(Katzung, pp. 785–786)*

493. **(B)** All aminoglycosides can produce ototoxicity, and this adverse reaction is most likely in the elderly, patients receiving high doses, patients receiving continuous therapy for longer than 5 days, and patients with renal insufficiency. *(Katzung, p. 785)*

494. **(D)** High doses of aminoglycosides can produce a neuromuscular blockade that results in respiratory paralysis. The paralysis can usually be reversed by prompt administration of calcium gluconate or neostigmine. *(Katzung, p. 786)*

495. **(E)** The most serious toxic effect of streptomycin is vestibular dysfunction accompanied by vertigo and loss of balance. This effect tends to be irreversible. *(Katzung, p. 787)*

496. **(A)** Aminoglycosides include streptomycin, kanamycin, amikacin, gentamicin, tobramycin, and others. *(Katzung, p. 784)*

497. **(D)** The combination enhances uptake of gentamicin due to inhibition of cell wall synthesis by the penicillin or vancomycin. *(Katzung, p. 788)*

498. **(E)** Neomycin is not well absorbed from the GI tract and is used in preparation for elective bowel surgery to reduce aerobic bowel flora while producing minimal blood levels or systemic toxicity. *(Katzung, pp. 790–791)*

499. **(D)** Gentamicin and tobramycin are both aminoglycosides with similar antimicrobial activities and virtually identical pharmacokinetic properties. They are effective against both gram-positive and gram-negative organisms and are generally given intravenously or intramuscularly because of poor absorption from the GI tract. *(Katzung, pp. 787–790)*

500. **(D)** Concentration-dependent killing means that the higher the concentration of drug, the greater the killing effect. Postantibiotic effect refers to the fact that bacterial killing persists for a significant amount of time after measurable levels of the aminoglycoside have disappeared. Toxicity of aminoglycosides tends to depend on the time that the drug concentrations are above a certain threshold level, although the threshold level may not be precisely defined. *(Katzung, p. 789)*

501. **(A)** The structure of sulfonamides most closely resembles the structure of PABA. They inhibit bacterial growth by blocking folic acid synthesis, which is essential for the production of purines and synthesis of nucleic acids. *(Katzung, pp. 793–794)*

502. **(D)** Sulfonamides inhibit the growth of both gram-positive and gram-negative bacteria by interfering with the formation of dihydrofolic acid, which is essential for production of purines and the synthesis of nucleic acids. *(Katzung, p. 793)*

503. **(D)** Resistance to sulfonamides can be caused by any of the three mechanisms listed in this item. *(Katzung, p. 793)*

504. **(C)** Sulfadoxine has a half-life of 7 to 9 days. The other sulfonamides listed in this item have short or intermediate half-lives measured in hours. *(Katzung, p. 795)*

505. **(E)** Intravenous trimethoprim–sulfamethoxazole is the agent of choice for moderately severe to severe pneumocystis pneumonia, especially in immunocompromised patients. Oral administration of this combination is also effective against many types of infection. *(Katzung, p. 796)*

506. **(C)** Sulfadiazine, like other orally effective sulfonamides, is widely distributed to bodily tissues and fluids, including the brain and CSF. *(Katzung, pp. 793–794)*

507. **(E)** Sulfadoxine is a long-acting, orally effective sulfonamide that is excreted slowly by the kidney due to high protein binding and extensive tubular reabsorption. *(Katzung, p. 794)*

508. **(E)** Intestinal microflora split sulfasalazine into sulfapyridine and 5-aminosalicylate (5-ASA). 5-ASA has an anti-inflammatory effect that is beneficial in ulcerative colitis, enteritis, and other inflammatory bowel disease. Because it releases 5-ASA in the intestine, sulfasalazine has a therapeutic effect similar to olsalazine, a dimer of 5-ASA, but it may not be as well tolerated. *(Katzung, pp. 794–795)*

509. **(E)** All of the agents listed in this item are derivatives of sulfonamides and are cross-allergenic with them. Other cross-allergenic agents include bumetanide, torsemide, and diazoxide. *(Katzung, p. 795)*

510. **(C)** Nephrotoxicity due to large doses of sulfadiazine is caused by precipitation of the drug, resulting in crystals in the urine. Since the drug is more soluble at alkaline than acid pH, sodium bicarbonate may be given to reduce the crystalluria. *(Katzung, p. 795)*

511. **(E)** Because trimethoprim is a weak base of $pK_a = 7.2$, it concentrates in prostatic fluid and vaginal fluid, which are more acid than plasma. *(Katzung, p. 796)*

512. **(C)** As a consequence of its antifolate activity, trimethoprim can produce megaloblastic anemia, leukopenia, and granulocytopenia. Use of folinic acid can prevent the hematologic toxicity caused by the combination of trimethoprim and sulfamethoxazole, but its use has been associated with increased morbidity and treatment failures in AIDS patients being treated with trimethoprim–sulfamethoxazole for pneumocystis pneumonia. *(Katzung, p. 797)*

513. **(D)** All three mechanisms of resistance listed in this item are known to occur in bacteria. Resistance most commonly results from trimethoprim-resistant dihydrofolate reductase encoded by plasmids. *(Katzung, p. 796)*

514. **(C)** Ciprofloxacin is a fluoroquinolone with excellent activity against gram-negative bacteria and moderate to good activity against gram-positive bacteria. *(Katzung, p. 797)*

515. **(A)** Nalidixic acid itself can be used for treatment of lower urinary tract infections, but it does not achieve systemic antibacterial levels. *(Katzung, p. 797)*

516. **(E)** Ciprofloxacin is a fluoroquinolone. This group of antibiotics inhibits bacterial topoisomerase II (DNA gyrase) and topoisomerase IV, thereby interfering with DNA synthesis. *(Katzung, p. 797)*

517. **(A)** All of the fluoroquinolones in this group have excellent activity against gram-negative bacteria, but ciprofloxacin is the most active against these organisms, especially *Pseudomonas aeruginosa*. *(Katzung, p. 797)*

518. **(C)** Fluoroquinolones are extremely well tolerated with the most common adverse effects being GI symptoms. Headache, dizziness, insomnia, skin rash, or abnormal liver function tests are observed occasionally. *(Katzung, p. 800)*

519. **(D)** Elevated levels of theophylline accompanied by an increased risk of adverse effects, especially seizures, can be caused by concomitant administration of theophylline and fluoroquinolones. *(Katzung, p. 800)*

520. **(A)** The five first-line agents for treatment of tuberculosis are: isoniazid, rifampin, pyrazinamide, ethambutol, and streptomycin. *(Katzung, pp. 803–804)*

521. **(D)** Isoniazid promotes the excretion of pyridoxine, which leads to a relative pyridoxine deficiency that causes the peripheral neuropathy observed in isoniazid-treated patients. *(Katzung, p. 806)*

522. **(D)** The antimycobacterial activity of rifampin is due to its strong binding to the beta subunit of bacterial DNA-dependent RNA polymerase, which inhibits the enzyme. Resistance is usually caused by one of several possible point mutations in the gene *(rpoB)* encoding for the beta subunit, resulting in prevention of binding. *(Katzung, p. 806)*

523. **(E)** Ethambutol causes a retrobulbar neuritis resulting in loss of visual acuity and red–green color blindness. *(Katzung, p. 807)*

524. **(C)** Pyrazinamide is converted by mycobacterial pyrazinamidase to pyrazinoic acid, which is the active form of the drug. The drug has greater activity against tubercle bacilli at acid pH than at neutral pH. It is taken up by macrophages and exerts its antimycobacterial action mainly against organisms in the acidic intracellular environment. *(Katzung, p. 807)*

525. **(B)** Isoniazid is a prodrug that is converted to its active form by mycobacterial catalase-peroxidase. In its activated form, the drug forms a covalent complex with an acyl carrier protein (AcpM) and a beta-ketoacyl carrier protein synthetase (KasA), resulting in inhibition of mycolic acid synthesis. *(Katzung, pp. 803–804)*

526. **(A)** Ethambutol inhibits mycobacterial arabinosyl transferases which are involved in the polymerization reaction of arabinoglycan. *(Katzung, p. 807)*

527. **(E)** Nearly all patients treated with clinically significant doses of amphotericin B suffer renal impairment. There are reversible and irreversible components of this toxicity. The reversible component is associated with decreased renal perfusion. The irreversible component is caused by renal tubular injury. *(Katzung, pp. 815–816)*

528. **(A)** The amphotericin B molecule may be described as having a double bond–rich side and a hydroxyl-rich side. The double bond–rich side binds to membrane lipids forming the outside of pores, and the hydroxyl-rich side of the drug molecule forms the inside lining of pores in the cell membrane, thus altering cell permeability. *(Katzung, p. 815)*

529. **(C)** Once inside the fungal cell, flucytosine is converted first to 5-fluorouracil, then to 5-fluorodeoxyuridine monophosphate, which inhibits DNA synthesis, and to fluorouridine triphosphate, which inhibits RNA synthesis. *(Katzung, pp. 816–817)*

530. **(E)** Terbinafine inhibits the fungal enzyme squalene epoxidase, thus interfering with the synthesis of ergosterol, and causing accumulation of squalene, which is toxic to the organism. *(Katzung, p. 820)*

531. **(A)** Amphotericin B is poorly absorbed from the intestine and is given by IV injection for treatment of systemic disease. It is widely distributed to most tissues, but it is poorly distributed in the CSF. *(Katzung, pp. 814–815)*

532. **(A)** The lipid vehicle reduces nonspecific binding of amphotericin B to mammalian membranes, thereby reducing the nephrotoxicity of the drug. *(Katzung, p. 815)*

533. **(A)** Acyclovir is an acyclic guanosine derivative that is phosphorylated by multiple steps within the cell to form the triphosphate. The nucleotide analog inhibits DNA synthesis in two ways: (1) It competes with deoxyGTP for the viral DNA polymerase, and (2) it causes chain termination when it is incorporated into the viral DNA. *(Katzung, p. 824)*

534. (D) Acyclovir is activated by phosphorylation to the triphosphosphate, and the nucleotide analog then interferes with DNA synthesis catalyzed by viral DNA polymerase. The first phosphorylation step, yielding the monophosphate, is catalyzed by viral thymidine kinase. Alteration of viral thymidine kinase appears to be the main mechanism of the development of resistance to the drug, and a second mechanism involves alteration of viral DNA polymerase. *(Katzung, pp. 824–825)*

535. (D) Both ganciclovir and zidovudine can cause myelosuppression and the toxic effect may be additive when both drugs are administered concomitantly. *(Katzung, pp. 829, 841)*

536. (C) Probenecid must be administered together with IV cidofovir to block active renal tubular secretion and thereby decrease the nephrotoxicity caused by cidofovir. *(Katzung, p. 829)*

537. (C) Fomivirsen inhibits cytomegalovirus replication by an antisense mechanism. The drug is an oligonucleotide that binds to target mRNA, resulting in inhibition of protein synthesis. *(Katzung, p. 830)*

538. (C) Zidovudine is a deoxythymidine analog that inhibits HIV-1 reverse transcriptase and can also be incorporated into the growing viral DNA chain, causing termination of the chain. *(Katzung, p. 831)*

539. (E) Didanosine is relatively contraindicated in patients with chronic alcoholism or other risk factors for pancreatitis. *(Katzung, pp. 833–834, 841)*

540. (E) The peripheral neuropathy associated with zalcitabine can be treatment limiting in 10 to 20% of patients. The neuropathy appears to be slowly reversible if the drug is withdrawn promptly. *(Katzung, p. 835)*

541. (B) Ritonavir is a potent inhibitor of the CYP3A and CYP2D6 isoforms of cytochrome P450 and thus interacts with numerous other drugs. In addition, plasma levels of ritonavir are decreased by drugs that induce the CYP3A isoform. *(Katzung, pp. 838–839)*

542. (B) CSF penetration of indinavir ranges as high as 76% of serum levels. *(Katzung, p. 839)*

543. (E) Both drugs inhibit uncoating of the virion by targeting the M2 protein within the membrane. *(Katzung, p. 840)*

544. (D) Didanosine is a nucleoside reverse transcriptase inhibitor. These agents competitively inhibit HIV-1 reverse transcriptase. They also can be incorporated into the growing viral DNA chain, thereby terminating the chain. *(Katzung, pp. 831–833)*

545. (C) Saquinavir and ritonavir are both protease inhibitors. Saquinavir is extensively metabolized by first-pass effect as it passes through the liver, thereby reducing the levels of drug that reach the systemic circulation. Ritonavir potently inhibits the cytochrome P450 isoform that metabolizes saquinavir (CYP3A4), resulting in less saquinavir being removed by first-pass metabolism and more reaching the systemic circulation. *(Katzung, pp. 838–839)*

546. (D) Metronidazole effectively eradicates intestinal and extraintestinal tissue infections by *E. histolytica*. Iodoquinol, diloxanide furoate, and paromomycin sulfate are effective for therapy of luminal infections, but not extraintestinal tissue infections by this organism. Mefloquine is used for therapy against chloroquine-resistant strains of *P. falciparum*, not *E. histolytica*. *(Katzung, pp. 893–896)*

547. (E) Trimethoprim and sulfamethoxazole block sequential steps in the metabolism of folic acid and thereby produce synergistic effects against *P. carinii* and other organisms. *(Katzung, pp. 795–797, 897)*

548. (E) The phosphate salt of chloroquine is well absorbed from the GI tract, and the drug is well distributed to most tissues. It is generally well tolerated. The emergence of resistant strains of *P. falciparum* since the 1940s has compromised the drug's utility in the treatment of malaria. It is the drug of choice against sensitive strains. *(Katzung, pp. 882–886)*

549. (D) Most antimalarial drugs do not eradicate the dormant liver forms of *P. vivax* and *P. ovale*, and therefore common therapy includes chloroquine to eradicate erythrocytic forms and primaquine to eradicate liver forms of these parasites. *(Katzung, p. 889)*

550. (D) Pyrimethamine and proguanil inhibit dihydrofolate reductase. Each of these drugs may be used in combination with a sulfonamide or sulfone, which inhibits dihydropteroate synthase, another enzyme in the folate pathway. *(Katzung, pp. 890–891)*

551. (A) Metronidazole has a disulfiram-like effect so that if alcohol is ingested during therapy, nausea and vomiting could result. *(Katzung, p. 895)*

552. (A) Cell cycle–nonspecific agents include: alkylating agents, antibiotics, cisplatin, and nitrosoureas. Cell cycle–specific agents include: antimetabolites, bleomycin peptide antibiotics, podophyllin alkaloids, and plant alkaloids. *(Katzung, p. 926)*

553. (A) P-glycoprotein is a cell surface transport molecule that expels a variety of foreign molecules from the cell and is responsible for multidrug resistance in cancer cells. *(Katzung, pp. 926–927)*

554. (E) Toxic reactions to alkylating agents include nausea and vomiting of CNS origin and toxicity in rapidly growing tissues such as bone marrow, GI tract, and gonads. The major toxicity is suppression of myelopoiesis, resulting in a fall in white blood cell count. Erythrocyte counts are affected to only a minor extent due to the long life span of these cells. *(Katzung, pp. 927–930)*

555. (B) Adjuvant chemotherapy with the regimens given as examples in this item are of most benefit in stage II with one to three pos-

itive lymph nodes. Women with stage II and involvement of four or more lymph nodes receive less benefit, and therapy for women with stage III and stage IV cancer is a major problem. *(Katzung, p. 951)*

556. (E) Approximately 95% of the patients described in this item respond to combination chemotherapy, and approximately 90% enter into complete remission. It appears that over half of those patients that enter complete remission are cured. *(Katzung, p. 952)*

557. (E) Cell cycle–specific agents include: antimetabolites, bleomycin peptide antibiotics, podophyllin alkaloids, and plant alkaloids. Cell cycle–nonspecific agents include: alkylating agents, antibiotics, cisplatin, and nitrosoureas. *(Katzung, p. 926)*

558. (D) Polyglutamate derivatives of methotrexate have greater inhibitory activity against enzymes involved in folate metabolism and are retained longer in cells than methotrexate. *(Katzung, p. 932)*

559. (A) Cyclophosphamide, chlorambucil, and other alkylating agents cause cell death mainly as a result of the transfer of their alkyl groups to various cellular constituents, nuclear DNA perhaps being the most important target. *(Katzung, pp. 926–927)*

560. (A) Cytarabine (Ara-cytosine) is converted in the body to Ara-CTP, which acts as a competitive inhibitor of DNA polymerase, thereby blocking DNA synthesis without directly blocking RNA or protein synthesis. *(Katzung, p. 935)*

561. (E) Vinblastine binds specifically to the microtubular protein tubulin and causes depolymerization of the microtubules that form the mitotic spindle. The result is arrest of mitosis in the metaphase. *(Katzung, pp. 935–936)*

562. (C) Etoposide and teniposide are drugs that form a ternary complex of the drug, DNA, and topoisomerase II, resulting in DNA damage through strand breakage. *(Katzung, p. 937)*

563. **(A)** Dactinomycin binds tightly to double-stranded DNA, resulting in interference with RNA synthesis. Ribosomal RNA synthesis is the most sensitive to the blockade, and this results in blockade of protein synthesis. *(Katzung, pp. 938–939)*

CHAPTER 7

Immunopharmacology
Questions

DIRECTIONS (Questions 564 through 576): Each of the numbered items or incomplete statements in this section is followed by answers or by completions of the statement. Select the ONE lettered answer or completion that is BEST in each case.

564. Which of the following classes of drugs represent drugs that are used for immunosuppression in transplant patients?

    (A) antiproliferative/antimetabolic agents
    (B) calcineurin inhibitors
    (C) glucocorticoids
    (D) all of the above
    (E) none of the above

565. Which of the following pharmacologic agents binds to cyclophilin, forming a complex that inhibits calcineurin in T lymphocytes?

    (A) azathioprine
    (B) cyclosporine
    (C) daclizumab
    (D) mycophenolate mofetil
    (E) sirolimus

566. Which of the following drugs binds to the intracellular protein, FK506-binding protein-12 (FKBP-12), forming a complex that leads to inhibition of T-lymphocyte activation and proliferation downstream from the interleukin-2 (IL-2) and other T-cell growth factor receptors?

    (A) azathioprine
    (B) basiliximab
    (C) mycophenolate mofetil

    (D) sirolimus
    (E) tacrolimus

567. Which of the following drugs binds to FKBP-12, forming a complex that leads to inhibition of calcineurin?

    (A) azathioprine
    (B) basiliximab
    (C) methylprednisolone
    (D) mycophenolate mofetil
    (E) tacrolimus

568. Which of the following statements is (are) true of antithymocyte globulin used as an immunosuppressive agent?

    (A) Anti-antibodies that develop in the patient limit the repeated use of this agent.
    (B) It is a monoclonal antibody preparation.
    (C) It selectively targets the CD3 receptor.
    (D) all of the above
    (E) none of the above

569. Which of the following agents is commonly administered prior to treatment with muromonab-CD3 in order to suppress the cytokine release syndrome?

    (A) basiliximab
    (B) daclizumab
    (C) glucocorticoids
    (D) all of the above
    (E) none of the above

570. Which of the following is a chimeric anti-tumor necrosis factor-alpha (anti-TNF-α) monoclonal antibody?

(A) basiliximab

(B) daclizumab

(C) etanercept

(D) infliximab

(E) none of the above

571. Which of the following is a molecule that downregulates immune responses?

(A) CD28

(B) CD80

(C) CD86

(D) CD152

(E) CD154

572. Which of the following pharmacologic agents appears to restore depressed immune function of B and T lymphocytes, monocytes, and macrophages?

(A) azathioprine

(B) levamisole

(C) mycophenolate mofetil

(D) sirolimus

(E) tacrolimus

573. Which of the following immune-modulating agents carries the strongest warning against its use in women who may become pregnant?

(A) cyclosporine

(B) levamisole

(C) sirolimus

(D) tacrolimus

(E) thalidomide

574. Use of which of the following pharmacologic agents has been linked to serious cardiovascular toxicity due to capillary leak syndrome?

(A) human recombinant IL-2

(B) interferon-alpha-2b

(C) interferon-beta-1a

(D) interferon-gamma-1b

(E) levamisole

575. Which of the following pharmacologic agents is most effective in causing activation of phagocytes and production of oxygen metabolites that are toxic to microorganisms?

(A) dexamethasone

(B) interferon-alpha-2b

(C) interferon-beta-1a

(D) interferon-gamma-1b

(E) prednisone

576. How long does the protection from passive immunization using an immune globulin preparation typically last?

(A) 1 to 3 days

(B) 1 to 3 weeks

(C) 1 to 3 months

(D) 1 to 3 years

(E) > 3 years

Answers and Explanations

564. **(D)** All of the drug classes listed in this item have been found to be useful for maintenance immunotherapy and treating acute immune rejection of organ transplants. *(Hardman et al., pp. 1464–1465)*

565. **(B)** The cyclophilin–cyclosporine complex inhibits Ca^{2+}-stimulated dephosphorylation of the cytoplasmic component of the nuclear factor of activated T lymphocytes (NFAT). Ordinarily, calcineurin dephosphorylates the cytoplasmic component of NFAT, enabling this cytoplasmic component to translocate to the nucleus. In the nucleus, the cytoplasmic component complexes with nuclear components, forming a combination that is required for activation of T-cells including transactivation of lymphokine genes. Inhibition of the calcineurin-catalyzed dephosphorylation of the cytoplasmic component of NFAT blocks T-cell activation in response to specific antigenic stimulation. *(Hardman et al., pp. 1466–1467)*

566. **(D)** The sirolimus-FKBP-12 complex inhibits the mammalian kinase, target of rapamycin (mTOR). Inhibition of mTOR blocks transition from the G_1 to the S phase of the cell cycle. *(Hardman et al., p. 1470)*

567. **(E)** The tacrolimus-FKBP-12 combination forms a complex with calcium, calmodulin, and calcineurin resulting in inhibition of calcineurin's phosphatase activity. Ordinarily, calcineurin dephosphorylates the cytoplasmic component of NFAT, enabling this cytoplasmic component to translocate to the nucleus. In the nucleus, the cytoplasmic component of NFAT complexes with nuclear components, forming a combination that is required for activation of T cells, including transactivation of lymphokine genes. Inhibition of the calcineurin-catalyzed dephosphorylation of the cytoplasmic component of NFAT blocks T-cell activation in response to specific antigenic stimulation. *(Hardman et al., pp. 1467–1469)*

568. **(A)** Antithymocyte globulin is a polyclonal antibody preparation that binds to many cell-surface antigens on T lymphocytes. Its repeated use is limited by the development of anti-antibodies in the patient. *(Hardman et al., pp. 1472–1473)*

569. **(C)** Administration of glucocorticoids prior to treatment with muromonab-CD3 greatly reduces the release of cytokines and the accompanying reactions. *(Hardman et al., p. 1474)*

570. **(D)** Infliximab appears to be useful for treatment of selected cases of rheumatoid arthritis and Crohn's disease. Etanercept also binds to TNF-α, but, rather than being a monoclonal antibody, it is a fusion protein made up of the ligand-binding region of the human TNF-α receptor and the Fc region of human IgG_1. *(Hardman et al., p. 1475)*

571. **(E)** CD154 downregulates an immune response by interacting with CD80 and CD86. *(Hardman et al., p. 1476)*

572. **(B)** Levamisole is used in selected patients with colon cancer, but its use has been linked to agranulocytosis, which has proved fatal in some cases. *(Hardman et al., p. 1477)*

573. **(E)** Although thalidomide use has been linked to severe, life-threatening birth defects, with appropriate precaution against its use in women who are or who may become pregnant, it is sometimes used to treat erythema nodosum leprosum. *(Hardman et al., p. 1477)*

574. **(A)** Capillary leak syndrome is associated with a decrease in vascular tone and leak of plasma proteins and fluid from the blood vessels into the extravascular space. *(Hardman et al., p. 1478)*

575. **(D)** Interferon-gamma-1b appears to differ from the other available interferons in its ability to stimulate phagocytes. *(Hardman et al., p. 1478)*

576. **(C)** Passive immunization involves the introduction of preformed antibodies to a patient who is about to be exposed to an antigen or who is already exposed. *(Hardman et al., pp. 1478–1479)*

CHAPTER 8

Toxicology
Questions

577. Toxicology is concerned with adverse effects of chemicals. Because there are a large number of possibly toxic compounds, various groups have established terminology to identify safe levels of exposure to these compounds. In occupational toxicology or environmental toxicology, the term used to define effects of a toxic agent on a population is

    (A) ADI—acceptable daily limit
    (B) ecotoxicology
    (C) TLV-C—threshold limit values for any time
    (D) TLV-STEL—threshold limit values for short-term exposure
    (E) TLV-TWA—threshold limit values for time-weighted average in a normal 8-hour workday

578. Air pollution is a concern of many individuals as cities become more and more technology driven. The most abundant pollutant in the atmosphere is

    (A) carbon monoxide
    (B) hydrocarbons
    (C) nitrogen oxides
    (D) ozone
    (E) sulfur oxides

579. Toxicity to which of the following agents is most likely due to its metabolism to free radicals?

    (A) benzene
    (B) carbon monoxide
    (C) nicotine
    (D) paraquat
    (E) pyrethrum

580. The presence of this toxicant results in the inability of oxygen-binding sites of hemoglobin to release oxygen to the tissues.

    (A) benzene
    (B) carbon monoxide
    (C) halogenated hydrocarbons
    (D) ozone
    (E) sulfur dioxide

581. Farmers or workers who deal with silage can be poisoned by which of the following inhaled agents?

    (A) carbon dioxide
    (B) nitrogen oxide
    (C) ozone
    (D) sulfur dioxide
    (E) toluene

582. Which of the following is a bluish irritant gas?

    (A) carbon dioxide
    (B) nitrogen oxide
    (C) ozone
    (D) sulfur dioxide
    (E) toluene

583. Which of the following types of botanical poisoning usually involves seizures as well as allergic responses, resulting in contact dermatitis?

    (A) dioxane
    (B) nicotine
    (C) paraquat
    (D) pyrethrum
    (E) rotenone

584. In which of the following compounds is the salt not readily absorbed through the skin but the base is?

    (A) dioxane
    (B) nicotine
    (C) paraquat
    (D) pyrethrum
    (E) rotenone

585. The group of compounds associated with liver, renal, and cardiac toxicity is

    (A) aromatic hydrocarbons
    (B) botanical insecticides
    (C) halogenated hydrocarbons
    (D) herbicides
    (E) organophosphate insecticides

586. Treatment of beta-adrenergic receptor blocker intoxication is accomplished by administration of

    (A) beta agonists
    (B) atropine
    (C) glucagon
    (D) intravenous (IV) fluids

587. The mnemonic DUMBELS refers to poisoning with

    (A) atropine
    (B) calcium channel blockers
    (C) carbon monoxide
    (D) digoxin
    (E) organophosphate insecticides

588. Theophylline intoxication is best managed by

    (A) beta agonists
    (B) beta antagonists
    (C) activated charcoal
    (D) anticonvulsants
    (E) sedative hypnotic administration

589. A common cause of suicide attempts is tricyclic drug overdose. This condition should be managed by

    (A) a dopamine infusion
    (B) administration of ammonium chloride to increase pH
    (C) administration of norepinephrine to raise blood pressure
    (D) Physostigmine to reverse anticholinergic side effects
    (E) Quinidine for suppression of arrhythmias

DIRECTIONS (Questions 590 through 601): Each group of questions in this section consists of groups of lettered headings followed by lists of numbered words or phrases. For each numbered word or phrase, select the ONE lettered heading that is most closely associated with it. Each lettered heading may be selected once, more than once, or not at all.

Questions 590 through 593

Match each agent with the appropriate clinical use.

    (A) deferoxamine
    (B) dimercaprol
    (C) edetate calcium disodium
    (D) penicillamine
    (E) succimer
    (F) trientine

590. Utilized primarily for the treatment of lead intoxication

591. Considered the first-line treatment for Wilson's disease

592. Administered intravenously or intramuscularly for the treatment of iron poisoning

593. Also known as British Anti-lewisite

Questions 594 through 598

Match the appropriate agent with its potential toxicity.

   (A) acetylcysteine
   (B) atropine
   (C) ethanol
   (D) naloxone
   (E) oxygen
   (F) pralidoxime

594. Carbon monoxide poisoning

595. Methanol poisoning

596. Opioid overdose

597. Early stages of organophosphate intoxication

598. Acetaminophen toxicity

Questions 599 through 601

Match each usage with the appropriate agent.

   (A) activated charcoal
   (B) cathartics
   (C) dialysis
   (D) emesis
   (E) gastric lavage

599. Used to enhance the elimination of iron tablets, enteric-coated agents, illicit drug packages

600. Should be avoided in patients who have ingested a petroleum distillate

601. May be useful in eliminating toxic compounds by a process called "gut dialysis"

Answers and Explanations

577. **(B)** TLV terminology relates to occupational toxicology, while ADI refers to environmental toxicology. Ecotoxicology is concerned with populations rather than individuals. *(Katzung, pp. 987–988)*

578. **(A)** By far, carbon monoxide is the greatest pollutant, accounting for 52% of air pollution. Sulfur oxides (14%), hydrocarbons (14%), nitrogen oxides (14%), and ozone (minor) are far less than carbon monoxide. *(Katzung, p. 989)*

579. **(D)** Paraquat accumulates in the body. After oral ingestion, the first signs may relate to the gastrointestinal system; however, within a few days, respiratory distress appears. This may progress to hepatic, renal, or cardiac involvement. *(Katzung, p. 996)*

580. **(B)** The binding affinity of carbon monoxide for hemoglobin is 220 times that of oxygen. Carboxyhemoglobin cannot transport oxygen, nor can the hemoglobin already combined with oxygen, release that oxygen to tissues. *(Katzung, p. 990)*

581. **(B)** The exposure of farmers to NO_2 in the silo can lead to deep lung irritation and pulmonary edema. Levels as low as 100 ppm can result in death. *(Katzung, p. 991)*

582. **(C)** Ozone is important in the earth's atmosphere because it absorbs ultraviolet light. It is an irritant to mucous membranes and when inhaled causes lung irritation. *(Katzung, p. 991)*

583. **(D)** A combination of compounds known as pyrethrum (six pyrethrins) is not very toxic to humans but when large amounts are absorbed they cause seizures and contact dermatitis. *(Katzung, p. 995)*

584. **(B)** Nicotine, a botanical insecticide, is extremely toxic as the alkaloid. A drop may be lethal when it is absorbed through the skin. However, the salt is not absorbed. *(Katzung, p. 994)*

585. **(C)** The agents used for general anesthesia, chloroform in particular, were well known for causing arrhythmias, kidney toxicity, and liver toxicity. *(Katzung, p. 992)*

586. **(C)** Administration of beta agonists, atropine, or IV fluids is generally ineffective. Glucagon, which can raise cyclic adenosine monophosphate (cAMP) levels by a mechanism that does not involve the beta-adrenergic receptor, is more effective. *(Katzung, p. 1020)*

587. **(E)** Diarrhea, urination, miosis and muscle weakness, bronchospasm, excitation, lacrimation and seizures, sweating, and salivation make up the signs and symptoms of organophosphate intoxication. Peripheral effects due to muscarinic receptor activation are treated with atropine. Pralidoxime may be somewhat helpful for other effects, but it does not penetrate the central nervous system (CNS). *(Katzung, p. 1021)*

588. **(B)** Theophylline inhibits phosphodiesterase enzymes and raises cAMP levels. Beta antagonists, especially propranolol, are effective in managing this intoxication. Activated char-

coal helps, but anticonvulsants and sedative–hypnotics are generally ineffective. *(Katzung, p. 1023)*

589. **(C)** The administration of norepinephrine is the most appropriate choice from the list given. Dopamine will not help (nerve endings are depleted and uptake inhibited), physostigmine will reverse the anticholinergic symptoms but will aggravate the depressed cardiac conduction and will also cause seizures. Sodium bicarbonate may help ammonium chloride has no effect. *(Katzung, p. 1023)*

590. **(C)** Other metals are chelated by the calcium disodium salt, but its primary use is for lead toxicity. It has no utility in the treatment of atherosclerotic cardiovascular disease. *(Katzung, p. 1008)*

591. **(D)** Copper accumulation can be eliminated with this agent; however, considerable toxicity is observed with penicillamine: hypersensitivity, nephrotoxicity, pancytopenia, and pyridoxine deficiency. *(Katzung, p. 1008)*

592. **(A)** Patients taking this agent should be warned that excretion in the urine will result in an orange-red color. Parenteral administration is the norm since bound iron (iron-carrying proteins) do not compete favorably with biologically chelated iron (microsomes, mitochondrial cytochromes). *(Katzung, p. 1009)*

593. **(B)** Dimercaprol was developed to counter the warfare agent know as lewisite, an arsenic containing gas. It is approved for use in the treatment of arsenic and mercury poisoning as the sole agent. It does have a high incidence of adverse side effects. *(Katzung, p. 1007)*

594. **(E)** Carbon monoxide combines reversibly with hemoglobin, and the most effective treatment is 100% oxygen by high-flow nonrebreathing mask. *(Katzung, pp. 990, 1018)*

595. **(C)** A loading dose of ethanol will compete with methanol for oxidation and lower the toxic by-products of methanol poisoning. The newer agent fomepizole may be effective. *(Katzung, pp. 392–393, 1018)*

596. **(D)** The standard treatment for patients suspected of having narcotic overdose is naloxone. This agent cannot be given without danger because acute withdrawal could be precipitated. Reversal of symptoms is evidence of opioid use. *(Katzung, p. 1018)*

597. **(F)** Before the organophosphate "ages," these highly reactive reactivators can compete with the organophosphate for the cholinesterase, thus reactivating the enzyme. This agent is known as PAM. *(Katzung, pp. 115, 1018)*

598. **(A)** Acetylcysteine will act as a glutathione substitute and bind the toxic metabolite as it is being produced. *(Katzung, pp. 1018–1019)*

599. **(B)** Cathartics like GoLYTELY or other balanced polyethylene glycol-electrolyte solutions may be helpful. *(Katzung, p. 1016)*

600. **(D)** Syrup (not extract) of ipecac is used for emesis in children but should be avoided with corrosive agents or petroleum-based compounds. *(Katzung, pp. 1016–1017)*

601. **(A)** There is a fair amount of questioning about the effectiveness of activated charcoal, administered in a ratio of 10:1 (charcoal to toxin). However, the large amount of charcoal may aid in eliminating toxic compounds through the gut ("gut dialysis"). *(Katzung, p. 1016)*

Nonsteroidal Analgesics and Gout
Questions

**DIRECTIONS (Questions 602 through 610): Each
of the numbered items or incomplete statements
in this section is followed by answers or by completions of the statement. Select the ONE lettered
answer or completion that is BEST in each case.**

602. A 4-year-old boy is seen in your office. His
mother has brought him in because he is very
warm. The intake notes indicate he has a
temperature of 103° F. He attends kinder-
garten, and there have been a large number
of upper respiratory infections at the site he
attends, most of them of viral origin. The
most appropriate approach would be to

    (A) administer a COX-2 inhibitor to avoid
    gastric irritation in this youngster
    (B) do nothing—the infection will run its
    course in a week
    (C) give acetaminophen for its antipyretic
    effect
    (D) place him in a lower-temperature water
    bath to assure that the temperature
    comes back into the normal range
    (E) recommend that he take a small dose of
    aspirin to control temperature

603. Your patient has been reading in the local
press that nonsteroidal anti-inflammatory
drugs (NSAIDs) are useful in preventing
heart attacks, and he wishes to obtain something to take advantage of this beneficial
drug action. He has had a long-standing
problem with gastric irritation from any
spicy food and has hemophilia. What advice
would you give?

    (A) Acetaminophen lacks the gastrointesti-
    nal (GI) irritation effect but is very effec-
    tive in inhibiting platelet aggregation.
    (B) He would probably be best served by
    not taking any drugs since the risk out-
    weighs the benefit.
    (C) Low-dose aspirin will do the "job" and
    will not cause upset like the full dose
    would.
    (D) Take one of the new COX-2 inhibitors;
    they are expensive but will not cause GI
    upset.
    (E) Use buffered aspirin since this will elim-
    inate the gastric irritation.

604. Which of the following statements about aspirin is correct?

    (A) Aspirin will block the generation of
    prostacyclin, thus removing a protective
    prostaglandin.
    (B) High doses of aspirin may exacerbate
    pain in patients with rheumatoid arthri-
    tis.
    (C) The antiplatelet action of aspirin is re-
    versible and wears off in about 6 to 8
    hours.
    (D) Visceral pain is effectively managed
    with aspirin.
    (E) While aspirin produces excellent analge-
    sia and antipyresis, it is not very effec-
    tive as an anti-inflammatory.

605. Aspirin intoxication causes a sequential set of complications, ranging from gastric intolerance to renal and respiratory failure. The production of metabolic acidosis would be considered

(A) lethal

(B) mild intoxication

(C) moderate intoxication

(D) severe intoxication

(E) therapeutic

606. In attaining relief from headache, which of the following forms of aspirin would be therapeutically superior?

(A) buffered aspirin

(B) concomitant use of H_2 blockers

(C) concomitant use of misoprostol

(D) enteric-coated aspirin

(E) none of the above, use regular aspirin

607. Ibuprofen

(A) causes GI irritation equivalent to aspirin

(B) has anti-inflammatory potency equivalent to aspirin

(C) is eliminated unchanged in the urine

(D) is not anti-inflammatory in doses recommended for over-the-counter purchase

(E) may effectively potentiate the action of aspirin

608. Many advertising claims have been made about the NSAIDs; however, in reviewing the pharmacodynamics of these compounds

(A) all NSAIDs except the COX-2 inhibitors irreversibly inhibit platelet aggregation

(B) NSAIDs, with the exception of aspirin, are reversible inhibitors of COX

(C) patients with kidney disease should select a non-nephrotoxic NSAID

(D) some of the NSAIDs do not cause gastric irritation

(E) the NSAIDs should be selected on the basis of analgesic versus antipyretic activity

609. In the treatment of rheumatoid arthritis, cyclosporine

(A) is considered a DMARD (disease-modifying antirheumatic drug)

(B) increases the levels of interleukin-2 (IL-2) and tumor necrosis factor-alpha (TNF-α)

(C) is a cyclo-oxygenase inhibitor with considerable toxicity

(D) use is based on greater anti-inflammatory action than NSAIDs

(E) usually acts fairly rapidly (within a week)

610. With regard to the treatment of rheumatoid arthritis with gold preparations

(A) clinical response, if it is going to appear, usually occurs within the first week of therapy

(B) it is most likely due to the action of gold to alter the functional capabilities of macrophages

(C) it is most often discontinued because of the ineffectiveness of this somewhat controversial approach

(D) patients tolerate the injections well since this compound is relatively nontoxic

(E) this insoluble compound can be administered only by injection

DIRECTIONS (Questions 611 through 616): Each group of questions in this section consists of groups of lettered headings followed by lists of numbered words or phrases. For each numbered word or phrase, select the ONE lettered heading that is most closely associated with it. Each lettered heading may be selected once, more than once, or not at all.

Questions 611 through 616

Match each description with the appropriate agent.

(A) allopurinol

(B) aspirin

(C) colchicine

(D) indomethacin

(E) probenecid

(F) sulfinpyrazone

611. This agent decreases the formation of uric acid by inhibiting xanthine oxidase.

612. Many individuals must discontinue this agent due to abdominal pain and diarrhea.

613. Indomethacin or colchicine should be administered in the early stages of treatment with this agent to prevent gouty arthritis episodes.

614. This agent is an organic acid originally designed to inhibit the excretion of penicillin.

615. This agent is often used in the initial treatment of gout as a prostaglandin synthase inhibitor.

616. This agent is an inhibitor of microtubular polymerization.

Answers and Explanations

602. **(C)** The best approach would be to recommend acetaminophen since it will lower temperature without the potential to cause Reye's syndrome. There is no need to take drastic action (the water bath). The COX-2 inhibitor is not indicated for simple temperature reduction; however, this temperature should be lowered. *(Katzung, pp. 603, 615)*

603. **(B)** While low-dose aspirin or buffered aspirin might seem a reasonable choice, this patient should not take any antiplatelet agents. COX-2 inhibitors and acetaminophen are not antiplatelet agents and would not be beneficial. *(Katzung, pp. 603, 615)*

604. **(A)** Administration of misoprostol, a prostaglandin E, derivative, is deemed beneficial in preventing ulceration. Its antiplatelet action is irreversible, it is a good anti-inflammatory, and it is used in high doses (2 to 3 g/d) to manage the pain of arthritis. *(Katzung, pp. 601–602)*

605. **(C)** The complications of aspirin toxicity increase from gastric irritation as follows: tinnitus, central hyperventilation, metabolic acidosis, vasomotor collapse, renal/respiratory failure to death. *(Katzung, p. 602)*

606. **(E)** The is little evidence that any of the choices provide a superior product when it comes to therapeutic efficacy. Enteric coating, while expensive, may decrease some gastritis, but H_2 blockers or buffering do not help. Misoprostol is cost effective in several groups of patients such as those with bleeding disorders, but it is very expensive and may cause diarrhea. *(Katzung, p. 602)*

607. **(D)** Ibuprofen causes less GI irritation, has greater anti-inflammatory potency (2x) and is completely metabolized by CYP2C8 and CYP2C9. The use of ibuprofen and aspirin together has been reported to decrease the total anti-inflammatory effect. *(Katzung, p. 605)*

608. **(B)** Aspirin irreversibly inhibits platelet cyclo-oxygenase; the other NSAIDs reversibly inhibit this enzyme. All NSAIDs (except the COX-2 selective agents) cause some gastric irritation. They are all potentially nephrotoxic, and all are analgesic, anti-inflammatory, and antipyretic. *(Katzung, pp. 598–599)*

609. **(A)** The use of toxic agents is based on the fact that NSAIDs relieve the inflammation and pain but do not modify the course of the disease. These agents, which act over months, are employed with the intent of arresting the progression of the disease process. *(Katzung, pp. 608–609)*

610. **(B)** The use of gold for the treatment of arthritis is controversial but some patients who can tolerate the toxicity (the major reason for dropout) may obtain a positive clinical response after several months of treatment. The mechanism of effect is unknown, but the most widely accepted mechanism seems to be inhibition of macrophage function. *(Katzung, pp. 610–611)*

611. **(A)** The inhibition of uric acid formation by enzyme inhibition decreases the urate pool and increases xanthine and hypoxanthine levels. *(Katzung, p. 619)*

612. **(C)** Colchicine, in addition to causing abdominal cramping, causes troublesome diarrhea in patients. *(Katzung, p. 617)*

613. **(A)** Allopurinol may cause acute attacks of gouty arthritis as tissue levels of urate crystals are being removed from tissues. The treatment prevents these gouty episodes. *(Katzung, p. 619)*

614. **(E)** Probenecid inhibits the secretory transporter in the proximal tubule so that the net reabsorption of uric acid is decreased. *(Katzung, p. 618)*

615. **(D)** Indomethacin and other prostaglandin synthase inhibitors also inhibit urate crystal phagocytosis. *(Katzung, p. 617)*

616. **(C)** The binding of colchicine to intracellular protein tubulin prevents its polymerization and thus inhibits leukocyte migration and phagocytosis. *(Katzung, p. 616)*

Gastrointestinal Pharmacology
Questions

617. A 30-year-old man who works as a financial advisor has been under a great deal of pressure by clients because of the declining stock market. He has been using antacids and large amounts of aspirin for indigestion and pain, respectively. He fears that he has developed an ulcer. Diagnostic studies confirm that he has a gastric ulcer. Which of the following statements is correct regarding this patient?

    (A) Antacids are particularly effective in inhibiting peptic ulcers, and he should continue their use at a higher dose or switch to a liquid preparation.

    (B) Combination therapy that includes an H_2 receptor antagonist and a proton pump inhibitor (PPI) should be instituted.

    (C) Combination therapy that includes an H_2 receptor blocker and antacids should be instituted.

    (D) H_2 receptor antagonists should be avoided because they are not effective in reducing the food-induced secretion of gastric acid.

    (E) Proton pump inhibitors are superior to H_2 receptor antagonists and to misoprostol in the healing of nonsteroidal anti-inflammatory drug (NSAID)-induced ulcers.

618. Proton pump inhibitors (PPIs)

    (A) act reversibly to inhibit the transport enzyme

    (B) are prodrugs and must be converted to the active compound

    (C) inhibit Na^+/K^+ adenosine triphosphatase (ATPase)

    (D) must enter the cell, since they act on the inside of the membrane

    (E) require an alkaline environment and are administered with bicarbonate

619. The most important determinant of the rate of healing of duodenal ulcers is

    (A) inhibition of prostaglandin production

    (B) suppression of nocturnal acid secretion

    (C) the amount of histamine produced

    (D) the balance between constipation and diarrhea induced by antacids

    (E) the protective effect of sucralfate

620. Antiemetic agents are generally known for their effect to inhibit chemically induced nausea and vomiting by acting on

    (A) H_1 receptors

    (B) H_2 receptors

    (C) serotonin receptors

    (D) the chemoreceptor trigger zone (CTZ)

    (E) the vomiting center

621. A 55-year-old man underwent a procedure in which damage to the vagus occurred. This resulted in reduced gastric emptying. An agent that would be effective in restoring motility is

(A) cimetidine

(B) hydroxyzine

(C) loperamide

(D) metoclopramide

(E) misoprostol

622. In the treatment of gastric upset with histamine antagonists, which of the following agents would be expected to alter drug metabolism?

(A) cimetidine

(B) famotidine

(C) nizatidine

(D) ranitidine

623. A 38-year-old woman is being treated with high doses of morphine for breast cancer, which has metastasized widely. She is in the terminal stages of life, and there is concern that she will not be able to tolerate large doses of morphine due to its constipating effect. A reasonable approach would be to

(A) add dioctyl sodium sulfosuccinate to the therapeutic regimen

(B) administer metoclopramide

(C) do nothing—it is the price of pain relief

(D) increase her intake of a bulking agent such as bran

(E) reduce the morphine to levels that do not cause constipation

DIRECTIONS (Questions 624 through 631): Each group of questions in this section consists of groups of lettered headings followed by lists of numbered words or phrases. For each numbered word or phrase, select the ONE lettered heading that is most closely associated with it. Each lettered heading may be selected once, more than once, or not at all.

Questions 624 through 627

Match each use or side effect with the appropriate gastrointestinal (GI) agent.

(A) sulfasalazine

(B) magnesium-based antacids

(C) mineral oil

(D) cascara

(E) aluminum-based antacids

624. A common side effect of this agent is constipation.

625. This agent is used for laxation when stimulation of peristalsis is desired.

626. This agent is considered a therapeutic stool softener.

627. Inflammatory bowel disease is treated with this combination product containing salicylates.

Questions 628 through 631

Match each use with the appropriate agent.

(A) infliximab

(B) castor oil

(C) methyl cellulose

(D) dronabinol

(E) bismuth subsalicylate

628. A marijuana derivative used in the management of nausea

629. An inhibitor of tumor necrosis factor-alpha (TNF-α) for the management of Crohn's disease

630. A hydrophilic colloid used as a laxative

631. A mucosal protective agent

Answers and Explanations

617. **(E)** NSAID-induced ulcers are best healed by PPIs, when compared with misoprostol or H_2 receptor antagonists. Antacids are ineffective. Combinations listed in choice B or C are not useful and often antagonize each other. H_2 receptor antagonists are very effective in reducing food-induced production of gastric acid. *(Katzung, pp. 1066–1067)*

618. **(B)** An acid environment is required to convert the prodrug to the active compound. It acts on the external side of the cell membrane to inhibit H^+/K^+ ATPase. *(Katzung, p. 1067)*

619. **(B)** Suppression of nocturnal acid secretion by administering H_2 (histamine) blockers at bedtime promotes healing. Reducing the dose to one half for maintenance therapy prevents recurrence. *(Katzung, pp. 1066–1067)*

620. **(D)** Chemically induced nausea and vomiting is due to stimulation of receptors in a highly vascular area of the brain known as the chemoreceptor trigger zone (CTZ). Receptors of the histamine and serotonin type may be involved. *(Katzung, pp. 1069–1070)*

621. **(D)** Metoclopramide is a prokinetic agent that promotes GI motility. It is more selective than cholinomimetic agents like bethanechol. *(Katzung, pp. 1068–1069)*

622. **(A)** Among the H_2 antagonists that are used to inhibit gastric acid secretion, only cimetidine slows hepatic microsomal oxidase metabolism to any major extent. *(Katzung, p. 1067)*

623. **(A)** A stool softener such as dioctyl sodium sulfosuccinate (docusate) is often added to the regimen to prevent or lessen the constipating effect of opioids administered for cancer pain. *(Katzung, p. 1071)*

624. **(E)** Aluminum-based antacids are astringent and usually result in constipation; therefore, they are often combined with an antacid that produces diarrhea (magnesium based) so that there will be a balance between the two actions on the intestinal tract. *(Katzung, p. 1066)*

625. **(D)** Cascara, senna, and aloes liberate emodin alkaloids and will stimulate increased peristalsis in the colon 6 to 8 hours after ingestion. *(Katzung, p. 1070)*

626. **(C)** The agents that form emulsions (dispersion of fats in water or vice versa, like detergents) soften the stool and aid passage. This group of agents includes mineral oil, glycerin suppositories, and dioctyl sodium sulfosuccinate. *(Katzung, p. 1071)*

627. **(A)** 5-Aminosalicylic acid cannot be taken orally, so sulfasalazine, which combines sulfapyridine with 5-aminosalicylic acid through an azo bond, was developed. In the distal ileum and colon the bacteria break down the compound to release 5-aminosalicylic acid. *(Katzung, p. 1072)*

628. **(D)** Derivatives of marijuana like dronabinol are effective antiemetics in some patients. The mechanism may involve the receptors in the CTZ. *(Katzung, p. 1070)*

629. **(A)** The use of a monoclonal antibody directed against TNF-α represents a new approach to the treatment of inflammatory bowel disease. *(Katzung, p. 1073)*

630. **(C)** Methylcellulose, like agar and psyllium seed, has the same effect as saline cathartics (magnesium citrate). These agents distend the large intestine by holding water by osmotic force. The distention results in peristalsis and evacuation of the bowel. *(Katzung, p. 1071)*

631. **(E)** Bismuth subsalicylate, which is the active ingredient in Pepto-Bismol, acts by a combination of methods. The major one appears to be binding to an ulcer, thus protecting it from acid and pepsin. It is also postulated to stimulate mucous production, stimulate prostaglandin synthesis, and inhibit the action of pepsin. It is used in combination with metronidazole and tetracycline to cure ulcers where *Helicobacter pylori* is involved. *(Katzung, p. 1068)*

CHAPTER 11

Asthma, Antihistamines, and Smooth Muscle
Questions

DIRECTIONS (Questions 632 through 659): Each of the numbered items or incomplete statements in this section is followed by answers or by completions of the statement. Select the ONE lettered answer or completion that is BEST in each case.

632. Bronchial asthma is characterized by

    (A) decreased responsiveness to methacholine
    (B) high levels of immunoglobulin E (IgE) in the plasma of affected individuals
    (C) increased levels of antigen in the atmosphere
    (D) nonspecific bronchial hyperreactivity
    (E) specific hyperreactivity of the airways to antigens

633. Pharmacologic management of bronchial asthma

    (A) does not include the use of humanized monoclonal anti-IgE antibody
    (B) is rather uncomplicated since the introduction of "spacers" for inhalers
    (C) may require the use of "controller" drugs
    (D) requires the continual use of beta-adrenergic agonists
    (E) with antihistamines will prevent immediate bronchoconstriction

634. The basis for the use of inhaled corticosteroids in the treatment of asthma is based on the knowledge that

    (A) airway inflammation is linked to increased airway responsiveness

    (B) eosinophilia is the primary cause of the late response
    (C) muscarinic antagonists will effectively reduce bronchial smooth-muscle contraction
    (D) preventing acute bronchospasm will inhibit the last asthmatic response
    (E) the condition is due to nonadrenergic, noncholinergic pathways

635. Methylxanthines are widely used for the management of bronchial asthma in many areas of the world where cost is an important factor. Which of the following agents is usually employed therapeutically?

    (A) aminophylline
    (B) caffeine
    (C) dyphylline
    (D) theobromine
    (E) theophylline

636. The mechanism of action of methylxanthines has involved the proposal of all of the following EXCEPT

    (A) inhibition of adenosine receptors
    (B) inhibition of antigenic challenge resulting in reduction of CD4 and CD8 lymphocytes
    (C) inhibition of muscarinic receptors
    (D) inhibition of phosphodiesterase
    (E) modulation of adenyl cyclase activity

637. The use of theophylline

    (A) is limited due to poor absorption

    (B) may cause excessive daytime drowsiness

    (C) requires lower doses in children because they clear the drug slower

    (D) requires periodic monitoring of plasma levels

    (E) usually results in stable levels unless kidney function is deteriorating

638. The mechanism of action of cromolyn is

    (A) activation of beta-adrenergic receptors

    (B) blockade of muscarinic receptors

    (C) inhibition of delayed chloride channels

    (D) inhibition of mast cell mediator release

    (E) inhibition of phosphodiesterase

639. Nedocromil is administered

    (A) and is more effective in adolescents

    (B) for acute phase responses

    (C) in an attempt to replace corticosteroids since they are more effective

    (D) in sustained-release oral capsules

    (E) prophylactically

640. For the management of bronchial asthma, beta-adrenergic agonists

    (A) are most effective when administered orally

    (B) are dangerous due to cardiac stimulation caused by most agents

    (C) are more effective if longer-acting compounds like salmeterol are used for acute-phase responses

    (D) should be administered by nebulizer to obtain a more uniform dose

    (E) should be restricted to beta$_2$ selective agents

641. A unique feature of ipratropium that makes it useful in treating bronchial asthma is

    (A) its long duration of action

    (B) its oral effectiveness

    (C) the effect on the central nervous system (CNS)

    (D) the fact that it is a quaternary amine

    (E) the immediate effect to inhibit bronchospasm

642. In the clinical use of corticosteroids, the LEAST important adverse effect is

    (A) adrenal suppression

    (B) hoarseness

    (C) oral candidiasis

    (D) osteoporosis

    (E) slowed rate of growth

643. Corticosteroids have been shown to be effective in all of the following EXCEPT

    (A) bronchodilation

    (B) improved quality of life

    (C) inhibition of eosinophilic airway inflammation

    (D) reduction of bronchial reactivity

    (E) reduction of frequency of asthma exacerbations

644. Histamine can be antagonized by several mechanisms. Physiologic inhibition occurs with the administration of

    (A) cimetidine

    (B) cromolyn

    (C) epinephrine

    (D) fexofenadine

    (E) promethazine

645. H$_2$ receptors are similar to

    (A) acetylcholine receptors

    (B) alpha-adrenergic receptors

    (C) H$_1$ receptors

    (D) H$_3$ receptors

    (E) serotonin receptors

646. A 28-year-old graduate student has a great deal of trouble staying awake in class. He never had this problem before, but this

spring he has been bothered by high pollen counts and has been taking a number of over-the-counter (OTC) products for allergies. His problem is most likely due to

(A) a condition known as narcolepsy

(B) he really has no problem, he just needs to drink coffee or a cola drink

(C) the metabolism of antihistamines in the OTC products to active sedatives

(D) the penetration of antihistamines into the CNS

(E) using compounds with a long half-life

647. The importance of the antihistamine fexofenadine lies in the fact that it

(A) causes torsade de pointes

(B) has a short duration of action (4 to 6 hours)

(C) is metabolized to an active compound

(D) is nonsedating and does not cause cardiac arrhythmias

(E) should be avoided if the individual using it drinks grapefruit juice

648. The antihistamine promethazine is best known for its action as

(A) a local anesthetic

(B) a muscarinic-blocking agent

(C) a sedative

(D) an alpha-adrenergic-blocking agent

(E) an antiemetic

649. A distraught mother tells you that her 5-year-old daughter has been suffering from a runny nose due to a "cold." She gave her daughter what she thought was one of her antihistamine tablets to ease the symptoms and to help the child sleep. She is concerned because the child is "hyper." She thinks the wrong drug was in the bottle. The most likely explanation is

(A) antihistamines can cause excitation and convulsions in children

(B) she gave the child a second-generation antihistamine

(C) the bottle contained something that caused CNS excitation

(D) the drug was metabolized to a toxic stimulant

(E) this is an atropine-like side effect of the medication

650. Which of the following statements about H_2 blockers is correct?

(A) H_2 blockers only inhibit gastric acid secretion stimulated by gastrin.

(B) Most of the histamine (H_2) blockers also inhibit H_1 and H_3 receptors.

(C) Nizatidine inhibits contractile activity of the stomach.

(D) Ranitidine is the most potent and most effective H_2 blocker.

(E) The toxicity of these H_2 blockers is remarkably low.

651. A 56-year-old woman who has a history of angina pectoris for which she takes propranolol is suffering from recurrent headaches. These headaches are of the migraine type. She has a friend who had migraine headaches, and she wishes to obtain a prescription for the same substance since it was "a lifesaver" for her friend. The substance is sumatriptan. The correct approach in this case is to

(A) not prescribe sumatriptan for this patient

(B) give her a trial of the drug and reevaluate

(C) give the drug of choice for this patient, a $5-HT_1$ agonist

(D) provide her with the desired prescription

(E) treat with a serotonin antagonist

652. A 48-year-old banker is suffering from shortness of breath. He weighs 380 pounds and is 5 feet 10 inches tall. In his effort to lose weight he has entered numerous weight-loss plans, including prescription medication. In the process of attempting to lose weight it has become more and more difficult for him to engage in any physical activity. This was not a problem before. The most likely cause of his problem is

(A) a high-protein diet
(B) excessive use of a 5-HT antagonist
(C) he was probably taking amphetamines
(D) ingestion of phentermine
(E) the use of dexfenfluramine

653. Melatonin

(A) acts to inhibit monoamine oxidase (MAO)
(B) appears to regularize sleep patterns
(C) has direct hypnotic activity
(D) is a precursor of serotonin
(E) is located in the posterior pituitary

654. The intense CNS vasoconstrictive action of ergot alkaloids is due to stimulation of

(A) alpha-adrenergic receptors
(B) $5\text{-}HT_2$ receptors
(C) dopamine receptors
(D) muscarinic receptors
(E) nicotinic receptors

655. It is well established that ergot alkaloids cause intense vasoconstriction, leading to gangrene. These agents also cause a phenomenon known as

(A) beta-receptor blockade
(B) epinephrine reversal
(C) parturition
(D) reverse peristalsis
(E) uterine retroversion

656. Models of bronchial asthma characterized by airway hyperreactivity and pulmonary

edema have been employed to test pharmacologic agents. Which of the following is an example of a species that has extreme sensitivity to histamine?

(A) dog
(B) guinea pig
(C) human
(D) mouse
(E) subhuman primate

657. A 46-year-old man is complaining that he experiences generalized itching. He has no other disease process, appears healthy, and is looking for some relief from this very irritating problem. An appropriate agent to manage this condition is

(A) cyclizine
(B) diphenhydramine
(C) fexofenadine
(D) phenytoin
(E) ranitidine

658. The treatment of motion sickness is most effective when

(A) diphenhydramine is the sole agent
(B) promethazine is employed
(C) scopolamine is used prophylactically
(D) ephedrine is combined with an H_1 antagonist
(E) cyclizine or meclizine is used

659. One of the side effects of some antipsychotic agents is a parkinsonian-like tremor. This may be antagonized by the

(A) alpha receptor–blocking effect of promethazine
(B) anticholinergic effects of benztropine
(C) antihistaminic effects of diphenhydramine
(D) anti-serotonin effect of cyproheptadine
(E) inhibition of mediator release by epinephrine

DIRECTIONS (Questions 660 through 671): Each group of questions in this section consists of groups of lettered headings followed by lists of numbered words or phrases. For each numbered word or phrase, select the ONE lettered heading that is most clearly associated with it. Each lettered heading may be selected once, more than once, or not at all.

Questions 660 through 665

In the diagram below, indicate the letter associated with the agent or process listed below.

660. This phase of the process is inhibited or reduced by acute administration of sympathomimetic agents.

661. At this point the initiating agent is most likely methacholine.

662. The production of interleukin-4 (IL-4), IL-5, granulocyte macrophage colony-stimulating factor (GM-CSF), tumor necrosis factor (TNF), and/or transforming growth factor (TGF) occurs during this time period.

663. Histamine, prostaglandin D_2 (PGD_2), leukotriene C_4, and other agents are responsible for this phase.

664. IgE is binding to mast cells at this time.

665. Inhibition of this fall in FEV_1 occurs as a consequence of chronic pretreatment with inhaled glucocorticoids.

Questions 666 through 671

Match each description with the appropriate agent.

(A) albuterol
(B) aminophylline
(C) beclomethasone
(D) cromakalim
(E) cromolyn
(F) ipratropium
(G) nifedipine
(H) nitric oxide donors
(I) prednisone
(J) salmeterol
(K) zafirlukast
(L) zileuton

666. An activator of potassium channels

667. Inhibitor of leukotrienes at the receptor level

668. Plays an important role in aspirin-induced asthma

669. Mainly used in large doses for severe acute episodes of asthma

670. A lipoxygenase inhibitor

671. The long-acting agent of choice for management of nocturnal asthma

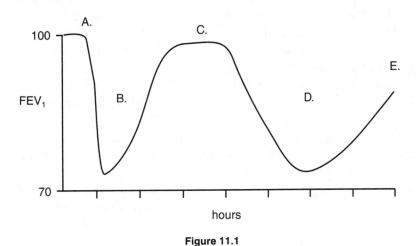

Figure 11.1

Answers and Explanations

632. (D) Bronchial asthma is quantified by measuring the fall in forced expiratory volume in one second (FEV_1) upon exposure to methacholine. This is to distinguish it from specific antigen-induced hyperresponsiveness. *(Katzung, p. 335)*

633. (C) Management of bronchial asthma includes the use of drugs that have an immediate effect to relax smooth muscle (short-term relievers) and the use of agents that prevent the response that occurs 2 to 8 hours later (long-term controllers). *(Katzung, pp. 333–334)*

634. (A) The acute bronchoconstriction and the late bronchoconstriction appear to be separate entities that are managed by different pharmacologic approaches. The use of corticosteroids is based on the knowledge that inhibition of inflammation prevents the development of airway hyperresponsiveness. *(Katzung, pp. 335, 343)*

635. (A) Aminophylline is the ethylenediamine salt of theophylline. It is used to improve solubility. Caffeine and theobromine present in coffee and cola beverages are virtually ineffective as bronchodilators. Dyphylline is a synthetic analog (shorter acting, less potent), and theophylline itself is rather insoluble. *(Katzung, p. 338)*

636. (C) Theophylline and its analogs have not been postulated to block muscarinic receptors. However, all of the other mechanisms have their proponents. *(Katzung, pp. 338–339)*

637. (D) Due to the potential adverse side effects, periodic monitoring is necessary. Changes in behavior due to liver disease or the addition of pharmacologic agents, which alter microsomal oxidase metabolism, require additional diligence. *(Katzung, pp. 339–340)*

638. (C) Until recently, the concept was that cromolyn and nedocromil inhibited mast cell release; however, new information has changed this view, and they are now thought to inhibit cellular activation by inhibiting delayed chloride channels in the cell membrane. *(Katzung, p. 337)*

639. (E) The use of cromolyn and nedocromil is limited to patients in whom it is shown to be effective by a trial of 4 weeks. It is used prophylactically and does not reverse the acute-phase response. Inhalation is the mode of administration and is most effective in children. *(Katzung, p. 337)*

640. (E) The beta$_2$ selective agents produce the least cardiac stimulation as long as low doses are administered. The most effective route of administration is by metered-dose inhaler since this route restricts the dose to the airway. Compounds like salmeterol and formoterol are long acting and not useful for acute episodes. *(Katzung, pp. 340–341)*

641. (D) Ipratropium is a charged nitrogen-containing compound. This charge limits its absorption and its action to the airway. It enhances the bronchodilation produced by adrenergic agonists. *(Katzung, p. 342)*

642. **(E)** The slogan used in most clinical conferences is that asthma can be lethal but shortened stature is not life threatening. Asthma itself, as a disease entity, has been shown to reduce height. *(Katzung, p. 343)*

643. **(A)** Corticosteriods do not directly cause bronchodilation but they do reduce reactivity and increase airway caliber. *(Katzung, p. 343)*

644. **(C)** Physiologic antagonism means that the body has mechanisms to counteract the effects of histamine. This process produces responses opposite to those of histamine but acting through separate receptors. *(Katzung, p. 269)*

645. **(E)** The receptors for histamine have been cloned. While H_2 receptors are similar to 5-HT_1 receptors, H_1 receptors are similar to muscarinic receptors. *(Katzung, p. 267)*

646. **(D)** Most OTC products contain first-generation antihistamines, which have sedation as a side effect. The sedation is due to the penetration of these compounds into the CNS. *(Katzung, pp. 270–271)*

647. **(D)** Fexofenadine is the metabolite of terfenadine. Terfenadine was a second-generation nonsedating antihistamine, which caused cardiac arrhythmias. It has been withdrawn from the market. *(Katzung, p. 270)*

648. **(E)** Promethazine, like most antihistamines of the first generation, has all of the effects noted; however, it is a widely used antiemetic. It is useful for prevention of motion sickness. *(Katzung, p. 273)*

649. **(A)** While it is not the most common side effect, antihistamines can and do cause excitation and even convulsions in children. The reason is not known. *(Katzung, p. 273)*

650. **(E)** Emptying time of the stomach is decreased due to contractility activity of nizatidine. This may be related to acetylcholinesterase inhibition. These agents block all phases of gastric acid secretion, and while their potency varies greatly, the effectiveness is relatively equal. Toxicity is remarkably low. *(Katzung, pp. 274–276)*

651. **(A)** Sumatriptan, a 5-HT_1 agonist, is contraindicated in patients with angina pectoris because these types of agents cause coronary artery vasospasm. *(Katzung, pp. 280–281)*

652. **(E)** It is likely that his problem results from the use of dexfenfluramine. This compound was found to cause valvular lesions, resulting in reduced cardiac output. *(Katzung, p. 281)*

653. **(B)** Melatonin, a serotonin metabolite, is located in the pineal gland. It is metabolized by MAO and regularizes sleep patterns. *(Katzung, p. 280)*

654. **(B)** Partial agonist action at alpha-adrenergic receptors accounts for some vasoconstriction. The effectiveness in migraine headache is thought to be related to serotonin receptor activation. *(Katzung, pp. 284–286)*

655. **(B)** The early studies of alpha-adrenergic receptors resulted in a reversal of the epinephrine vasoconstrictor response to that of a vasodilator (i.e., epinephrine reversal). This is due to the predominance of alpha receptors, which are activated at higher concentrations of epinephrine. When these receptors are blocked by ergot, the beta receptor vasodilator response predominates and blood pressure decreases. *(Katzung, p. 284)*

656. **(B)** Guinea pigs are known to be extremely sensitive to histamine. Human, dogs, mice, and subhuman primates react like the guinea pig when injected with pertussis vaccine. The analogy has been made between humans with asthma and guinea pig or humans following pertussis vaccination. *(Katzung, p. 268)*

657. **(B)** Of the agents given, all are antihistamines except phenytoin (its old name was diphenylhydantoin, which led to some confusion). The most commonly used agent for itching (pruritus) is diphenhydramine, one of the older H_1 antihistamines. It is commonly known by its trade name, Benadryl. *(Katzung, p. 273)*

658. (D) The antihistamines cause drowsiness, and the combination with ephedrine improves their effectiveness in prevention (prophylaxis) of motion sickness. *(Katzung, p. 273)*

659. (B) The anticholinergic effect of antihistamines like benztropine have been used to suppress the parkinsonian symptoms caused by other pharmacologic agents. *(Katzung, p. 272)*

660. (B) Adrenergic beta agonists selective for $beta_2$ receptors in airway smooth muscle are generally effective in reversing or inhibiting this reduction in FEV_1. *(Katzung, pp. 334–335)*

661. (A) The trigger for measuring FEV_1 is usually methacholine in increasing concentrations. *(Katzung, pp. 334–335)*

662. (C) Production of mediators of the inflammatory response precedes the late-phase reaction. *(Katzung, p. 334)*

663. (B) The fall in FEV_1 that occurs during the early phase and is reversed by sympathomimetic amines is due to histamine and related mediators released from the mast cell. *(Katzung, pp. 334–335)*

664. (A) In the antigen-mediated concept of asthma, it is binding of IgE to the mast cell that is responsible for the subsequent release of histamine. *(Katzung, p. 333)*

665. (D) The late-phase reaction that is due to mediators of inflammation is inhibited by glucocorticoids. The use of inhaled agents limits the adverse effect of these powerful anti-inflammatory agents. *(Katzung, pp. 334–335)*

666. (D) This compound in an investigational status directly hyperpolarizes smooth-muscle cells (potassium channels) and blocks alpha adrenoceptors. *(Katzung, p. 345)*

667. (K) Leukotrienes are generated by activation of the arachidonic acid pathway. Blocking the receptor for leukotriene D has been effective in inhibiting exercise-induced asthma. *(Katzung, p. 344)*

668. (K) Zafirlukast, the blocker of leukotriene D seems to be particularly effective in the 5 to 10% of asthmatics who are aspirin sensitive. *(Katzung, p. 344)*

669. (I) When urgent care is needed for severe asthma, prednisone or methylprednisolone is employed for short term (10 days). *(Katzung, p. 343)*

670. (L) The production of leukotrienes by the lipoxygenase pathway can be inhibited by zileuton, which was developed as an approach to inhibiting the leukotriene pathway. *(Katzung, p. 344)*.

671. (J) Salmeterol is not useful for acute management of asthma but is effective in preventing nighttime episodes. *(Katzung, p. 341)*

Practice Test
Questions

1. When doses of acetaminophen greatly exceed therapeutic levels, toxic metabolites can accumulate in the body because of the inability of the phase II reaction to convert the toxic metabolites to inactive products. The reason for the failure of the phase II reaction is the limited amount of one of the following compounds required for the reaction. Which compound is it?

   (A) acetyl coenzyme A (CoA)
   (B) glutathione
   (C) glycine
   (D) S-adenosylmethionine
   (E) uridine diphosphate (UDP) glucuronic acid

2. The danger in using partial agonists like pentazocine is that they

   (A) antagonize endogenous peptides and exaggerate pain responses
   (B) are not reliably reversed by naloxone
   (C) cause more severe respiratory depression than pure agents
   (D) produce hallucinations and nightmares
   (E) promote rapid eye movement (REM) and non–rapid eye movement (NREM) sleep

3. In treating patients with Parkinson's disease the effectiveness of levodopa therapy wanes due to

   (A) continuous loss of nigrostriatal neurons
   (B) increased responsiveness of cholinergic pathways
   (C) ineffectiveness of carbidopa
   (D) tachyphylaxis to dopamine
   (E) the lack of penetration of levodopa in the central nervous system (CNS)

4. In a pregnant patient with a history of asthma, complications occur during labor and delivery. A cesarean section is ordered. The anesthesiologist attempts to intubate the patient, and both heart rate and oxygen saturation begin to fall even though oxygen is being delivered to the patient. The proper drug to give is

   (A) atropine to restore heart rate
   (B) epinephrine to reverse the bronchospasm
   (C) lidocaine to prevent arrhythmias
   (D) thiopental to deepen the anesthesia and relieve stress.
   (E) tubocurarine to relax skeletal muscles and facilitate intubation

5. The use of ergot alkaloids or their derivatives is contraindicated in

   (A) hyperprolactinemia
   (B) induction of labor
   (C) migraine headache
   (D) postpartum hemorrhage
   (E) senile cerebral insufficiency

6. The duration of action of which of the following neuromuscular blocking agents would most likely be prolonged in patients who have an atypical variant of plasma cholinesterase that is inhibited only about 20% by dibucaine when the "dibucaine number" is determined under standardized conditions?

(A) atracurium
(B) mivacurium
(C) pancuronium
(D) rapacuronium
(E) vecuronium

7. Which of the following drugs is eliminated from the body mainly by excretion of the unchanged drug or its 3-hydroxy metabolite in the bile?

(A) atracurium
(B) cisatracurium
(C) mivacurium
(D) pancuronium
(E) vecuronium

8. Which of the following compounds is known to be more slowly metabolized in some individuals due to a reduced rate of hydroxylation caused by a genetic polymorphism of CYP2C19?

(A) acetaminophen
(B) dextromethorphan
(C) quinidine
(D) S-mephenytoin
(E) testosterone

9. Which of the following drugs would be most appropriate for treating the malignant hyperthermia triggered by a combination of general anesthesia and a neuromuscular blocking agent?

(A) carisoprodol
(B) chlorphenesin
(C) chlorzoxazone
(D) dantrolene
(E) orphenadrine

10. Ketamine produces a catatonic state with amnesia and analgesia. This is referred to as

(A) conscious sedation
(B) deep sedation
(C) dissociative anesthesia
(D) neuroleptanalgesia
(E) neuroleptanesthesia

11. What is the main mechanism whereby cimetidine alters the response to warfarin?

(A) It decreases the affinity of warfarin for vitamin K epoxide reductase.
(B) It enhances the metabolism of warfarin.
(C) It increases the affinity of warfarin for vitamin K epoxide reductase.
(D) It inhibits the metabolism of warfarin.
(E) It interferes with normal platelet function.

12. Which of the following is the most common dose-related adverse reaction to treatment with ethosuximide?

(A) diplopia
(B) drowsiness
(C) gastric distress
(D) leukopenia
(E) skin rashes

13. Many of the benzodiazepines are effective as anticonvulsants and skeletal muscle relaxants. An exception to this general effect is

(A) clonazepam
(B) diazepam
(C) flurazepam
(D) lorazepam
(E) zolpidem

14. Which of the following statements about tetracyclines is most accurate?

(A) They are bactericidal for many gram-positive and gram-negative bacteria.
(B) They are bactericidal for many gram-positive but not gram-negative bacteria.
(C) They are bacteriostatic for many gram-positive and gram-negative bacteria.

(D) They are bacteriostatic for many gram-negative but not gram-positive bacteria.

(E) They are bacteriostatic for many gram-positive but not gram-negative bacteria.

15. Which of the following neurologic reactions to antipsychotic agents typically appears after months or years of treatment and is manifest as involuntary, quick choreiform movements that may involve muscles of the face, eyelids, mouth, tongue, trunk, or limbs?

(A) acute dystonia

(B) akathisia

(C) neuroleptic malignant syndrome (NMS)

(D) parkinsonism

(E) tardive dyskinesia

16. The benzodiazepine that is known as the "date rape" drug is

(A) chloral hydrate

(B) flunitrazepam

(C) Mickey Finn

(D) secobarbital

(E) thiopental

17. In diabetic patients with renal disease, a particular benefit is obtained by treating with

(A) angiotensin-converting enzyme (ACE) inhibitors

(B) alpha-adrenergic-blocking agents

(C) angiotensin receptor blockers

(D) beta-adrenergic-blocking agents

(E) thiazides

18. A 34-year-old man presents with a syndrome resembling systemic lupus erythematosus (SLE). The drug most likely to cause the drug-induced condition is

(A) amiodarone

(B) procainamide

(C) quinidine

(D) tocainide

(E) verapamil

19. Digoxin toxicity may occur following antibiotics because

(A) about 10% of digoxin is metabolized by bacteria in the intestine, and antibiotics inhibit this process

(B) antibiotics change the membrane potential, and the result is increased absorption of digoxin

(C) digoxin is metabolized to a more lipid-soluble compound in the presence of antibiotics and thus more readily absorbed

(D) the structure of digoxin and antibiotics is similar, resulting in binding of digoxin to the antibiotic

(E) they both compete for similar binding sites, and antibiotics have a greater affinity for the site

20. The mechanism of action of calcium channel blockers is

(A) dependent on keeping the channel open and inhibiting repolarization

(B) dependent on the presence of T-type channels

(C) due to binding on the intracellular side of the channel

(D) mimicked by the action of brevetoxins, which act on the "h" gate within the channel

(E) similar to that of sodium channel blockers, which act on the extracellular side of the channel

21. Antidepressants have numerous uses, including treatment of

(A) aggressive behavior and delusional episodes

(B) enuresis and obsessive–compulsive disorders

(C) hypertension and constipation

(D) obesity and gregarious behavior

(E) urinary retention and acute pain

22. The effect of which of the following agents can be reversed by administration of protamine sulfate?

    (A) clopidogrel
    (B) eptifibatide
    (C) tirofiban
    (D) unfractionated heparin
    (E) warfarin

23. Which of the following urinary electrolyte patterns matches with the agent listed?

    (A) acetazolamide/high sodium
    (B) acetazolamide/low bicarbonate
    (C) furosemide/high sodium
    (D) hydrochlorothiazide/high bicarbonate
    (E) spironolactone/high potassium

24. Which of the following is the most appropriate route of administration of oxytocin used to enhance milk ejection in mothers who are breast feeding their babies?

    (A) intramuscular (IM) injection
    (B) intravenous (IV) infusion
    (C) nasal spray
    (D) oral administration
    (E) subcutaneous injection

25. What is the major complication of radio-iodine therapy for hyperthyroidism?

    (A) heart toxicity
    (B) hypothyroidism
    (C) kidney toxicity
    (D) liver toxicity
    (E) thyroid cancer

26. Which of the following changes in plasma lipids and lipoproteins is LEAST likely to be produced by estrogens?

    (A) decrease in apolipoprotein B (apo B) levels
    (B) decrease in high-density lipoprotein (HDL) levels
    (C) decrease in low-density lipoprotein (LDL) levels
    (D) decrease in total cholesterol levels
    (E) increase in triglyceride levels

27. Which of the following is the main mechanism of action of combination oral contraceptives?

    (A) change in motility and secretion in uterine tubes
    (B) change in the cervical mucus
    (C) change in the endometrium
    (D) inhibition of ovulation
    (E) stimulation of uterine contractility

28. Which of the following conditions represent(s) the most common toxic reaction(s) to metformin when used as a single antidiabetic agent?

    (A) gastrointestinal (GI) disturbances
    (B) hypertension
    (C) hypoglycemia
    (D) mental confusion and bizarre behavior
    (E) orthostatic hypotension

29. Which of the following vitamins can be used for the treatment of scurvy?

    (A) nicotinic acid
    (B) vitamin A
    (C) vitamin B_1 (thiamine)
    (D) vitamin C
    (E) vitamin D

30. What is the primary mechanism whereby probenecid raises blood levels of penicillins?

    (A) It blocks the uptake of penicillins into the CNS.
    (B) It decreases glomerular filtration rate.
    (C) It impairs tubular secretion of penicillins by the kidney.
    (D) It increases the rate of absorption of the penicillins.
    (E) It inhibits cytochrome P450 enzymes in the liver.

31. The abuse of cocaine produces a very intense dependence with a high relapse rate, which is thought to be due to the intense pleasure experienced by administering high concentrations of cocaine to the brain. The routes producing the fastest and highest blood levels of cocaine are

    (A) IV and oral
    (B) IV and smoking
    (C) nasal and IV
    (D) oral and smoking
    (E) smoking and nasal

32. What other antibiotics are usually used together with gentamicin sulfate against *Pseudomonas, Proteus, Enterobacter, Klebsiella, Serratia, Stenotrophomonas,* and other gram-negative rods?

    (A) beta-lactam antibiotics
    (B) macrolides
    (C) oxazoladinones
    (D) streptogramins
    (E) sulfonamides

33. The antimicrobial activity of trimethoprim is caused by its inhibition of which of the following bacterial enzymes?

    (A) dihydrofolate reductase
    (B) dihydropteroate synthase
    (C) enolpyruvate transferase
    (D) RNA polymerase
    (E) topoisomerase II and topoisomerase IV

34. Which of the following types of drugs is generally the most effective treatment for the acute dystonia caused by antipsychotic agents?

    (A) anticholinergic antiparkinsonian drugs
    (B) dantrolene and other muscle relaxants
    (C) ergot alkaloids
    (D) neuromuscular blocking agents
    (E) replacement of the offending agent with a more potent antipsychotic agent

35. Which of the following statements most accurately reflects the pharmacokinetics of ciprofloxacin?

    (A) After absorption, it is not distributed to most body fluids and tissues.
    (B) It is eliminated mainly by biliary excretion.
    (C) It is eliminated mainly by renal excretion.
    (D) It is extensively metabolized by liver enzymes to inactive products.
    (E) It is ineffective by the oral route.

36. Drug therapy is not always the most appropriate approach to treating hyperlipidemias. Which of the following conditions is first managed by dietary changes?

    (A) familial combined hyperlipoproteinemia
    (B) familial dysbetalipoproteinemia
    (C) familial hypercholesterolemia
    (D) familial hypertriglyceridemia
    (E) primary chylomicronemia

37. Which of the following mechanisms accounts for the antifungal activity of the azole drugs?

    (A) formation of pores in the cell membrane
    (B) inhibition of cytochrome P450 enzymes
    (C) inhibition of DNA and RNA synthesis
    (D) inhibition of ribosomal protein biosynthesis
    (E) inhibition of squalene epoxidase

38. Severe and life-threatening skin rashes have been reported during therapy with which of the following drugs?

    (A) efavirenz
    (B) indinavir
    (C) nevirapine
    (D) saquinavir
    (E) zidovudine

39. Which of the following adverse drug reactions is most closely associated with glucose-6-phosphate dehydrogenase (G6PD) deficiency?

    (A) angioedema
    (B) cinchonism
    (C) hemolysis
    (D) hypoglycemia
    (E) skin rashes

40. What is the most frequent second malignancy encountered in patients receiving cancer chemotherapy?

    (A) acute myelogenous leukemia (AML)
    (B) carcinoma of the breast
    (C) carcinoma of the thyroid gland
    (D) GI carcinomas
    (E) non-Hodgkin's lymphomas

41. Which of the following drugs binds to estrogen receptors and acts as a partial agonist inhibitor of estrogen in estrogen-sensitive tissues and tumor cells?

    (A) bleomycin
    (B) procarbazine
    (C) tamoxifen
    (D) topotecan
    (E) vincristine

42. Which of the following actions best represents a known effect of lipocortin?

    (A) inhibition of antibody production by B lymphocytes
    (B) inhibition of the killing of microorganisms by macrophages
    (C) inhibition of the production of prostaglandins and leukotrienes in macrophages, monocytes, endothelial cells, and fibroblasts
    (D) inhibition of the release of cytokines from lymphocytes, macrophages, and monocytes
    (E) inhibition of the release of histamine from basophils

43. Rattlesnake envenomation is managed by

    (A) administering large amounts of anti-venin
    (B) incision and suction
    (C) the use of ice packs
    (D) unnecessary motion
    (E) using tourniquets

44. Hemoperfusion or hemodialysis is NOT useful for intoxication due to

    (A) carbamazepine
    (B) procainamide
    (C) theophylline
    (D) tricyclic antidepressants (TCAs)
    (E) valproic acid

45. A patient presents to your office with signs and symptoms of gout. Upon taking a history, it is learned that he is taking "baby" aspirin for its antiplatelet action. Your treatment of this patient is to

    (A) administer allopurinol
    (B) begin the administration of probenecid to determine if this improves the symptoms
    (C) discontinue the aspirin since low doses inhibit uric acid secretion
    (D) not administer any medications, simply cut down on dietary purines to lower uric acid levels
    (E) start with low dose indomethacin as a prophylactic measure

46. Bronchial asthma responds to a variety of pharmacologic agents. Which group of patients is most likely to have a beneficial effect from muscarinic antagonists?

    (A) individuals requiring high doses of atropine
    (B) individuals with a high degree of vagal tone
    (C) patients in the midst of an acute asthmatic episode

(D) patients with mucus plugging

(E) those who have an established immunoglobulin E (IgE)-mediated response

47. Histamine activates a number of receptors. Which of the following is a correct statement regarding the action of histamine?

(A) H_1 receptor activation results in an increase in cyclic adenosine monophosphate (cAMP).

(B) Inositol phosphate is increased as a consequence of stimulating H_2 receptors.

(C) The activation of H_2 receptors is a G-protein coupled mechanism.

(D) The location of H_3 receptors is presynaptic.

(E) The stimulation of mast cell histamine release is an H_1 receptor mechanism.

48. Histamine antagonists were developed in the early 1930s, but these compounds were never able to inhibit the production of gastric acid in response to histamine. The reason is

(A) H_1 blockers were needed to inhibit this response

(B) H_3 receptor blockers were not available

(C) mepyramine had not been discovered yet

(D) the CNS depressant effect of the early antihistamines was not powerful enough

(E) the original antihistamines blocked H_1, not H_2, receptors

49. The adverse effects of theophylline in the management of respiratory diseases do NOT include

(A) cardiac arrhythmias

(B) CNS stimulation

(C) convulsions

(D) diaphragmatic contraction

(E) release of catecholamines

50. A 45-year-old dentist developed a hypersensitivity to local anesthetic agents because of his frequent exposure to them in his dental practice. He now needs dental work and is in serious need of a local anesthetic. What options are available?

(A) Employ an antihistamine with local anesthetic action.

(B) Give him thiopental intravenously.

(C) There are none—he will have to endure the pain.

(D) Use a general anesthetic agent such as halothane.

(E) Use an agent that provides topical anesthesia such as ethyl chloride spray.

Answers and Explanations

1. **(B)** Each of the compounds listed is a reactant in one of the phase II metabolic pathways. Glutathione is the reactant whose availability is exceeded by toxic amounts of acetaminophen. *(Katzung, pp. 56–58)*

2. **(D)** These compounds tend to produce nightmares and hallucinations. *(Katzung pp. 520–521)*

3. **(A)** The primary reason for loss of effectiveness is the continual disease progression with a continual loss of nigrostriatal neurons. *(Katzung, p. 465)*

4. **(B)** The oxygen saturation is falling due to irritation of the airways as a consequence of the attempted intubation. Epinephrine will relieve the bronchospasm and aid in restoring heart rate. *(Katzung, p. 130)*

5. **(B)** Ergot alkaloids or their derivatives are used for hyperprolactinemia (bromocriptine), migraine headache (ergotamine), and postpartum hemorrhage (ergonovine). Dihydroergotoxine has been tried for cerebral insufficiency; however, there is no evidence of benefit. These compounds should never be used for induction of labor or to induce abortion because they do not produce rhythmic contraction but rather a powerful spasm that results in both maternal and fetal death. *(Katzung, pp. 286–287)*

6. **(B)** When the "dibucaine number" is determined under standardized conditions, dibucaine inhibits normal plasma cholinesterase by about 80%, but atypical plasma cholinesterase by only about 20%. Since the duration of action of mivacurium is brief, mainly because it is rapidly hydrolyzed by plasma cholinesterase, patients with the atypical enzyme may manifest a prolonged neuromuscular blockade with this drug. *(Katzung, pp. 450–451)*

7. **(E)** Vecuronium is an intermediate-duration neuromuscular blocking agent with an approximate duration of action of 20 to 35 minutes. Eighty-five percent of an injected dose is excreted in the bile. *(Katzung, p. 450)*

8. **(D)** S-mephenytoin is the (S) stereoisomer of the anticonvulsant mephenytoin, which is normally hydroxylated in the 4 position of the phenyl ring prior to glucuronidation and excretion. Poor metabolizers appear to totally lack stereospecific S-mephenytoin hydroxylase activity due to genetic polymorphism and the drug may accumulate showing signs of sedation and ataxia in response to doses that are well tolerated in normal individuals. *(Katzung, pp. 59–60)*

9. **(D)** Malignant hyperthermia is a rare but very serious disorder caused by sudden and prolonged release of calcium from the sarcoplasmic reticulum, resulting in massive muscle contraction, lactic acidosis, and hyperthermia. Dantrolene interferes with the release of calcium from the sarcoplasmic reticulum, and is therefore useful for treating malignant hyperthermia. *(Katzung, pp. 459–460)*

10. **(C)** The term *dissociative anesthesia* is reserved for the action of ketamine. Neuroleptanalge-

sia is a combination of droperidol and fentanyl. The addition of nitrous oxide to neuroleptanalgesia results in neuroleptanesthesia. The terms *conscious* and *deep sedation* may be a combination of agents to provide drug-induced alleviation of anxiety and pain with an altered level of consciousness. The use of greater concentrations of agents results in a patient not easily aroused (deep). *(Katzung, pp. 432–433)*

11. **(D)** Cimetidine inhibits the metabolism of warfarin, often requiring a reduction of the warfarin dose in order to avoid overanticoagulation. *(Katzung, pp. 60–61)*

12. **(C)** The gastric distress can often be avoided by starting therapy with a low dose of ethosuximide and increasing the dosage gradually until therapeutic levels are achieved. *(Katzung, p. 409)*

13. **(E)** The nonbenzodiazepine, zolpidem, lacks anticonvulsant and skeletal muscle relaxant effects. *(Katzung, p. 374)*

14. **(C)** Tetracyclines are bacteriostatic and are effective against many gram-positive and gram-negative bacteria, including anaerobes, rickettsiae, chlamydiae, mycoplasmas, and L forms. *(Katzung, p. 776)*

15. **(E)** Tardive dyskinesia occurs more often in elderly than in young patients and may become worse upon withdrawal of the antipsychotic agent. Replacement of the offending agent with a more potent antipsychotic agent may help. *(Hardman et al., pp. 502–503)*

16. **(B)** Flunitrazepam (rohypnol, "roofies") is a tasteless, odorless compound that is placed in the drink of a victim, making the person unable to defend him- or herself or to remember what happened (amnesia). Thiopental is referred to as "truth serum," and chloral hydrate is the compound that combines with ethanol to produce the so-called Mickey Finn. *(Katzung, p. 537)*

17. **(A)** It has been demonstrated that the presence of concomitant disease is a reason for selecting a particular agent since both diseases may benefit from the treatment. This is the case with diabetic patients with renal disease. *(Katzung, p. 175)*

18. **(B)** As many as 33% of patients on long-term procainamide therapy develop reversible lupus-related symptoms. *(Katzung, p. 231)*

19. **(A)** The inhibition of bacteria reduces the bacterial conversion of digoxin to an inactive compound. Therefore, more is absorbed and greater toxicity may occur. *(Katzung, p. 203)*

20. **(C)** The calcium channel blockers used clinically are similar to sodium channel blockers in that they act on the intracellular side of the channel and are more effective when the channel is in the depolarized state. *(Katzung, p. 190)*

21. **(B)** Antidepressant agents have been successfully employed in managing obsessive–compulsive disorders, enuresis, chronic pain, bulimia, attention-deficit disorder, and panic disorder, in addition to depression. *(Katzung, pp. 505–506)*

22. **(D)** Protamine sulfate is administered intravenously to form a stable complex with heparin that has no anticoagulant activity. Excess protamine sulfate has anticoagulant activity of its own. *(Katzung, p. 569)*

23. **(C)** The large changes in urinary excretion occur as follows:

Carbonic anhydrase inhibitors—high bicarbonate
Loop diuretics—high sodium
Thiazides—moderate sodium, some increase in potassium
Potassium sparing—lower potassium and bicarbonate. *(Katzung, p. 260)*

24. **(C)** For use in lactating mothers, oxytocin is given by nasal spray. It is ineffective orally because it is broken down in the GI tract. For

induction of labor, it is usually given by IV infusion. *(Hardman et al., pp. 1558–1560)*

25. **(B)** The major complication of radioiodine therapy is hypothyroidism. This occurs in about 80% of the patients who are treated. *(Katzung, p. 655)*

26. **(B)** Estrogens increase plasma concentrations of HDL and triglycerides, whereas they decrease concentrations of cholesterol, LDL, and apo B. *(Katzung, pp. 683–685)*

27. **(D)** Contraception is produced mainly by inhibition of pituitary function and the resultant inhibition of ovulation. In cycles in which ovulation does occur, other effects may prevent pregnancy, namely, changes in the uterine endometrium, cervical mucus, and motility and secretion in the uterine tubes. *(Katzung, p. 693)*

28. **(A)** The most common toxic reactions to metformin are GI disturbances, which occur in up to 20% of patients. These include anorexia, nausea, vomiting, abdominal discomfort, and diarrhea. Metformin used as the sole antidiabetic agent does not cause hypoglycemia. *(Katzung, p. 728)*

29. **(D)** Scurvy results from vitamin C deficiency, and therefore vitamin C is used to treat this condition. *(Hardman et al., pp. 1769–1770)*

30. **(C)** Probenecid impairs the tubular secretion of weak acids, including beta-lactam antibiotics. *(Katzung, p. 759)*

31. **(B)** The administration of cocaine by inhaling the free base provides blood concentrations as rapidly and as high as IV administration. *(Katzung, pp. 538–539)*

32. **(A)** Gentamicin is often used together with beta-lactam antibiotics because of the synergistic effect against bacteria. The synergism is due in part to improved penetration of gentamicin into the cell due to inhibition of cell wall synthesis. *(Katzung, p. 788)*

33. **(A)** Trimethoprim inhibits dihydrofolate reductase, the enzyme that catalyzes the conversion of dihydrofolate to tetrahydrofolate, a step that is essential in the production of purines and synthesis of nucleic acids. The drug inhibits this enzyme in bacteria about 50,000 times more efficiently than it inhibits the same enzyme in mammalian cells. *(Katzung, p. 795)*

34. **(A)** Acute dystonia generally responds well to anticholinergic antiparkinsonian drugs administered by a parenteral route. *(Hardman et al., p. 501)*

35. **(C)** Like most fluoroquinolones, ciprofloxacin is eliminated from the body mainly by renal excretion. Dose adjustment is required for patients with renal impairment. *(Katzung, p. 799)*

36. **(E)** This condition is best managed without drug therapy. Marked restriction of total fat content in the diet provided effective treatment. *(Katzung, p. 585)*

37. **(B)** The azole drugs inhibit fungal cytochrome P450 enzymes, leading to a reduction in the synthesis of ergosterol, which is an essential component of the cell membrane. *(Katzung, p. 817)*

38. **(C)** Skin rash occurs in approximately 17% of patients receiving nevirapine and is dose limiting in approximately 7%. In some patients, skin rash has reportedly been severe and life threatening. Fulminant hepatitis has also been occasionally associated with therapy with this drug. *(Katzung, p. 836)*

39. **(C)** Primaquine, quinine, quinidine, and chloroquine may cause hemolysis or methemoglobinemia in people with G6PD deficiency. *(Katzung, pp. 883–890)*

40. **(A)** Some types of cancer chemotherapies are associated with second malignancy as a late complication. AML has been observed in patients receiving chemotherapy for Hodgkin's disease, breast carcinoma, multiple myeloma, and ovarian carcinoma. *(Katzung, pp. 955–956)*

41. **(C)** Due to its action at estrogen receptors, tamoxifen is useful for the treatment of breast cancer in patients who have tumors in which estrogen receptors or progesterone receptors can be demonstrated. *(Katzung, pp. 941–942)*

42. **(C)** Lipocortin is a protein that is induced by glucocorticoids, and which inhibits phospholipase A2, thereby interfering with the production of prostaglandins and leukotrienes. *(Hardman et al., pp. 1661–1662)*

43. **(A)** Unnecessary motion is useful, but the best treatment is antivenin. It may be necessary to administer large amounts of antivenin and to be prepared for an anaphylactic reaction. The other choices usually do more harm than good. *(Katzung, p. 1022)*

44. **(D)** TCAs, amphetamines, benzodiazepines, and other agents that have a large volume of distribution are not easily removed by dialysis-type processes. *(Katzung, pp. 1016–1017)*

45. **(C)** Low-dose aspirin will inhibit the secretory transporter for uric acid and increase uric acid levels. Simply eliminating aspirin may be an easily accomplished means of alleviating the symptoms. *(Katzung, p. 618)*

46. **(B)** Muscarinic antagonists are most effective when given to supplement other therapy and in a "group" or "subset" of patients who have increased parasympathetic activity. Low doses are effective and should be employed since high doses promote mucous plugging and tachycardia. *(Katzung, p. 342)*

47. **(D)** The pattern of receptor activation is:

    H_3 located presynaptically; G-protein coupled

    H_2 located in cardiac muscle, gastric mucosa, mast cells; cAMP

    H_1 located in smooth muscle; IP_3 *(Katzung, p. 267)*

48. **(E)** The early agents were H_1 blockers, and H_2 receptors or blockers were not known at that time. The H_2 blockers were required for inhibition of gastric acid secretion. *(Katzung, pp. 267, 274)*

49. **(D)** The effect on diaphragmatic performance is thought to account for the positive effect on ventilatory response in patients with irreversible airflow obstruction. *(Katzung, pp. 338–339)*

50. **(A)** Diphenhydramine and promethazine are actually more potent than procaine in their local anesthetic action and can be employed in patients with allergic responses to local anesthetic drugs. *(Katzung, p. 273)*

Bibliography

Hardman JG, Limbird LE, Gilman AG. *Goodman & Gilman's The Pharmacological Basis of Therapeutics,* 10th ed. New York: McGraw-Hill, 2001.

Katzung BG. *Basic and Clinical Pharmacology,* 8th ed. New York: McGraw-Hill, 2001.